Urgent and Out-of-Hours Primary Care

a practical guide for clinicians

Urgent and Out-of-Hours Primary Care

a practical guide for clinicians

UPDATED EDITION

H.K. Bhupal

MBBS MRCGP MRCP(UK) DRCOG DFSRH MFFLM PGDip(SEM)

GP Partner in Buckinghamshire

Scion

ISBN 9781914961588

First edition published in 2022 (ISBN 9781914961014)

A CIP catalogue record for this book is available from the British Library.

Scion Publishing Limited

The Old Hayloft, Vantage Business Park, Bloxham Road, Banbury OX16 9UX, UK

www.scionpublishing.com

Important Note from the Publisher
The information contained within this book was obtained by Scion Publishing Ltd from sources believed by us to be reliable. However, while every effort has been made to ensure its accuracy, no responsibility for loss or injury whatsoever occasioned to any person acting or refraining from action as a result of information contained herein can be accepted by the authors or publishers.

Readers are reminded that medicine is a constantly evolving science and while the authors and publishers have ensured that all dosages, applications and practices are based on current indications, there may be specific practices which differ between communities. You should always follow the guidelines laid down by the manufacturers of specific products and the relevant authorities in the country in which you are practising.

Although every effort has been made to ensure that all owners of copyright material have been acknowledged in this publication, we would be pleased to acknowledge in subsequent reprints or editions any omissions brought to our attention.

Registered names, trademarks, etc. used in this book, even when not marked as such, are not to be considered unprotected by law.

Readers are reminded that medicine is a constantly evolving science and that there may be specific practices which differ between communities. All dosages for medication are correct at the time of writing and are for adults; however, readers are advised to check the British National Formulary prior to prescribing any medication, to ensure the dosages are correct and up to date. You should always follow the guidelines laid down by the manufacturers of specific products and the relevant authorities in the country in which you are practising.

Feedback, errors and omissions

We are always pleased to receive feedback (good and bad) about our books – if you would like to comment on any of our books, please email info@scionpublishing.com.

We've worked really hard with the author to ensure that everything in the book is correct. However, errors and ambiguities can still slip through in books as complex as this. If you spot anything you think might be wrong, please email us and we will look into it straight away. If an error has occurred, we will correct it for future printings and post a note about it on our website so that other readers of the book are alerted to this.

Thank you for your help.

Typeset by Evolution Design & Digital Ltd, Kent, UK
Printed in the UK
Last digit is the print number: 10 9 8 7 6 5 4 3

Contents

Index of conditions

"Merely to have survived is not an index of excellence"
Anthony Hect

Index of conditions by symptom

"Symptoms, they are in reality nothing but the cry of suffering organs"
Jean Martin Charcot

Common presenting symptoms in OOH primary care and their acute causes (with least common causes shown at the end of each list).

- **Gastrointestinal**: gastro-oesophageal reflux disease, oesophageal rupture — *Chapter 11*
- **Musculoskeletal**: costochondritis, muscular strains, rib fractures — *Chapter 19*
- **Skin**: infections, shingles — *Chapter 17*
- **Anxiety** — *Chapter 15*

Dizziness

Determine if this is true vertigo or light-headedness

- **Acute and common causes of vertigo**:
  - **ENT**: labyrinthitis, acute vestibular neuritis, benign paroxysmal positional vertigo, Ménière's disease — *Chapter 18*
  - **Neurological:** subarachnoid haemorrhage, cerebrovascular accident — *Chapter 9*
- **Acute and common causes of light-headedness**:
  - (**Pre**)**syncope** — *Chapter 7*
  - **Hypoglycaemia** — *Chapter 10*
  - **Anxiety** — *Chapter 15*
  - **Drugs and alcohol (intoxication and withdrawal)** — *Chapter 16*

Earache

- **Ear conditions**: otitis externa, otitis media, barotrauma, foreign bodies, mastoiditis, Eustachian tube dysfunction — *Chapter 18*
- **Referred pain from the temporomandibular joint** — *Chapter 19*
- **Referred pain from dental pathology** — *Chapter 18*
- **Referred pain from oral and pharyngeal pathology** — *Chapter 18*
- **Trigeminal neuralgia** — *Chapter 9*
- **Herpes zoster** — *Chapter 17*
- **Temporal (giant cell) arteritis** — *Chapter 12*

Eye pain — *Chapter 14*

If the condition is causing pain or a drop in visual acuity, consider a referral to the on-call ophthalmologist

- **Peri-orbital conditions**: cellulitis, shingles, dermatitis
- **Corneal conditions**: corneal abrasions, corneal ulcers
- **Deep orbital structures**: orbital cellulitis, scleritis, uveitis, iritis, acute angle-closure glaucoma
- **Referred pain from ENT structures** — *Chapter 18*
- **Referred pain from dental pathology** — *Chapter 18*
- **Referred pain from neurological causes** — *Chapter 9*

Facial pain

- **Neurological**: headaches, trigeminal neuralgia — *Chapter 9*
- **Referred pain from ear pathology** — *Chapter 18*
- **Referred pain from temporomandibular joint pathology** — *Chapter 19*
- **Referred pain from dental pathology** — *Chapter 18*
- **Referred pain from oral and pharyngeal pathology** — *Chapter 18*
- **Trigeminal neuralgia** — *Chapter 9*
- **Herpes zoster** — *Chapter 17*
- **Temporal (giant cell) arteritis** — *Chapter 12*

- **Acute sinusitis** *Chapter 18*
- **Nasal infections** *Chapter 18*
- **Skin infections** *Chapter 17*
- **Peri-orbital and orbital cellulitis** *Chapter 14*

Headaches

- **Neurological**: migraines, tension-type headaches, subarachnoid haemorrhage, meningitis, neuralgia *Chapter 9*
- **Referred pain from dental pathology** *Chapter 18*
- **Referred pain from ENT pathology**: otitis media, mastoiditis, acute sinusitis, pharyngitis *Chapter 18*
- **Referred pain from eye pathology**: periorbital cellulitis, corneal injuries *Chapter 14*
- **Referred pain from temporomandibular joint dysfunction** *Chapter 19*
- **Tonsillitis**, Eustachian tube dysfunction *Chapter 18*
- **Endocrine**: diabetic ketoacidosis, hypoglycaemia *Chapter 10*
- **Hypertensive crises** *Chapter 7*
- **Temporal (giant cell) arteritis** *Chapter 12*
- **Pyrexia** *Chapter 22*

Pelvic pain

- **Urological**: cystitis, urinary tract infections, pyelonephritis, renal colic, acute urinary retention *Chapter 13*
- **Male genitalia**: testicular torsion, orchitis, epididymitis, prostatitis *Chapter 21*
- **Female genitalia**: pelvic inflammatory disease, ectopic pregnancy, pregnancy complications, endometriosis, endometritis, ovarian cyst rupture, ovarian cyst haemorrhage, ovarian cyst torsion and ovarian torsion *Chapter 20*

Shortness of breath

- **Cardiovascular**: acute coronary syndrome, angina, carditis (peri-, myo-, endo-), aortic dissection, left or biventricular impairment causing pulmonary oedema *Chapter 7*
- **Respiratory**: pulmonary embolism, pneumothorax, haemothorax, asthma, acute bronchitis, pneumonia, exacerbation of chronic obstructive pulmonary disease, pulmonary oedema, pleural effusion *Chapter 8*
- **Gastrointestinal**: oesophageal rupture *Chapter 11*
- **Musculoskeletal**: costochondritis, muscular strains, rib fractures *Chapter 19*
- **Sepsis** *Chapter 22*
- **Anxiety** *Chapter 15*
- **Severe pain** anywhere in the body

Syncope

- **Cardiovascular**: vasovagal, hypotension, arrhythmias, acute coronary syndrome *Chapter 7*
- **Neurological causes**: seizure, subarachnoid haemorrhage, cerebrovascular accident *Chapter 9*

Preface

"Live as if you were to die tomorrow, learn as if you were to live forever"

Mahatma Gandhi

This book has arisen from my interest in family medicine, general medical practice and urgent medical care. It stems from my experience working at the front end of these fields of medicine, as well as being involved in the commissioning, development, implementation and provision of urgent care services in England.

This book is aimed at doctors, medical students, nurses, paramedics, pharmacists and anyone who has an interest in out-of-hours primary care and urgent medical care. It deals with acute medical conditions, ailments and illnesses which a primary care clinician will be faced with when working outside a hospital setting and armed with only basic diagnostic aids.

I have always thought of a GP as being a 'true doctor', and I state this without any intention to disrespect my colleagues who specialise in one field of medicine. I relish the opportunity to treat patients of different ages and not limit myself to a particular area of the body or a specialty. Being able to deal with a multitude of problems, be it mental health issues or musculoskeletal problems, and being the first port of call for patients, is a privileged position to be in.

For me this is the true art of being a doctor; when on the edge and with limited access to diagnostic equipment a clinician is left with only his or her quick thinking and clinical skills to make rapid-fire diagnoses and develop and implement management plans for patients who may be, or could become very unwell. The old adage – that 80% of the time the diagnosis can be obtained from the history, 15% of the time from the examination and 5% of the time from investigations – still rings true.

My aim was to provide front-line healthcare professionals with a quick reference pocket book. Although not exhaustive, the intention was to cover the most common conditions seen in an out-of-hours primary care or urgent medical care setting.

As well as clinical conditions the book also contains my experiences of working as an out-of-hours General Medical Practitioner and the change in working towards remote consultations. It deals with the complexities and challenges of telephone triage and video consultations, as well as home visits.

Notes on some of the common medico-legal pitfalls are also included and tips on how these can be avoided.

Since the Covid-19 pandemic and the increased emphasis on remote consultations, the need to be able to diagnose and treat patients remotely is even greater. This book aims to provide the reader with the skills required to do this safely and effectively.

I have used icons to represent telephone, video and face-to-face consultations (see *Abbreviations*), thereby giving the reader an indication of which conditions can be managed remotely and via which format. In some situations a combination of the above may be required in order to assess and manage the patient. If enough information cannot be obtained remotely (via telephone or video consultation), then always consider a face-to-face consultation. Have a low threshold for assessing elderly patients and children face-to-face.

Red flag features are highlighted in red boxes, and key points are summarised at the end of each chapter. I have highlighted when an emergency ambulance should be arranged for the patient, along with which category.

In addition to this I have provided information on key features to look out for and when an admission to hospital is warranted.

Where possible I have tried to utilise images to assist the reader and clarify the text.

I have opened each chapter with a quote which I hope will be relevant to the chapter and will also interest and inspire, as well as amuse the reader.

Whilst every effort has been made to reference and credit original sources of information, I am more than happy to be corrected and to amend and acknowledge any information in subsequent editions.

All dosages for medication are correct at the time of writing and are for adults; however, I would advise the reader to check the British National Formulary prior to prescribing any medication, to ensure the dosages are correct and up to date.

To the readers of this book: I wish you all the best and good luck in your endeavours.

Hardeep Kumar Bhupal

Acknowledgements

"If I can touch the blue sky and feel the rays of the sun on my face, it is only because I am standing on the shoulders of giants."

Hardeep K. Bhupal

I would like to thank my wife Elizabeth for her support and my children Ambika, Abhijai and Aarav for always making me smile. I would like to thank my parents for channelling my endeavours into academia when I was a child; without their guidance I would not have achieved my ambition of being a doctor. I am grateful to my siblings Aman and Yogeeta for keeping me grounded. I would also like to thank Yogeeta and Ankit, both accomplished clinical pharmacists, for reviewing the dosages of medication in this book.

I would like to thank my teachers past and present who continue to inspire and motivate me.

I would like to thank Jonathan Ray, Clare Boomer and the team at Scion Publishing for their support and for believing in the viability of this book; I am eternally grateful.

I would also like to thank Dr David Lloyd and Dr Michael Ip, two respected and experienced colleagues with a wealth of knowledge in General Practice, for reviewing the manuscript.

Most importantly I would like to thank my patients; I have been privileged to listen to them, have their concerns shared with me, and been allowed to work with them so we can get through their troubles together.

About the author

"I've missed more than 9000 shots in my career. I've lost almost 300 games. 26 times, I've been trusted to take the game winning shot and missed. I've failed over and over and over again in my life. And that is why I succeed."

Michael Jordan

Dr Hardeep Kumar Bhupal went to school in west London; he graduated from the University of the West Indies in 2003. He has worked in Acute Medicine and Emergency Medicine departments in London and the south-east of England.

He has gained the following qualifications by examination:

MBBS	Bachelor of Medicine, Bachelor of Surgery
MRCGP	Member of the Royal College of General Practitioners
MRCP (UK)	Member of the Royal College of Physicians (UK)
DRCOG	Diplomate of the Royal College of Obstetricians and Gynaecologists
DFSRH	Diplomate of the Faculty of Sexual and Reproductive Health
MFFLM	Member of the Faculty of Forensic and Legal Medicine
PGDip (SEM)	Postgraduate Diploma in Sports and Exercise Medicine

He is currently a General Medical Practitioner in Chesham. In the past he has been clinical lead for urgent care in Enfield and Buckinghamshire. He has been involved in the development, implementation and provision of urgent medical care services in London and Buckinghamshire.

He works as an out-of-hours GP in urgent care in London, Buckinghamshire, Bedfordshire and Hertfordshire.

He is actively involved in education and is a GP registrar educator and medical student teacher. He is an author and examiner in Clinical Forensic and Legal Medicine and has worked as a physician in Clinical Forensic and Legal Medicine. He is a GP Appraiser for NHS England.

He also has a specialist interest in Sports and Exercise Medicine and in the past has worked with the medical team at Reading Football Club and provided medical cover to athletes at the Commonwealth Games in Glasgow.

He currently lives in Hertfordshire with his family.

The Declaration of Geneva

As a member of the medical profession:

"I solemnly pledge to dedicate my life to the service of humanity;
The health and well-being of my patient will be my first consideration;
I will respect the autonomy and dignity of my patient;
I will maintain the utmost respect for human life;
I will not permit considerations of age, disease or disability, creed, ethnic origin, gender, nationality, political affiliation, race, sexual orientation, social standing or any other factor to intervene between my duty and my patient;
I will respect the secrets that are confided in me, even after the patient has died;
I will practise my profession with conscience and dignity and in accordance with good medical practice;
I will foster the honour and noble traditions of the medical profession;
I will give to my teachers, colleagues, and students the respect and gratitude that is their due;
I will share my medical knowledge for the benefit of the patient and the advancement of healthcare;
I will attend to my own health, well-being, and abilities in order to provide care of the highest standard;
I will not use my medical knowledge to violate human rights and civil liberties, even under threat;
I make these promises solemnly, freely, and upon my honour."

World Medical Association (2021) *WMA Declaration of Geneva*.
www.wma.net/policies-post/wma-declaration-of-geneva

Abbreviations

This icon indicates that the condition can usually be assessed and managed via telephone.

This icon indicates a face-to-face consultation is recommended.

This icon suggests the use of a video consultation would be appropriate.

AC	ante cibum (before food)
BD	bis die (twice daily)
g	gram
IM	intramuscular
IV	intravenous
kg	kilogram
L	litre
mcg	microgram
mg	milligram
ml	millilitre
mm	millimetre
mmol/L	millimoles per litre
OD	omni die (every day)
OM	omni mane (every morning)
ON	omni nocte (every night)
OOH	out-of-hours
PC	post cibum (after food)
PO	per os (taken by mouth)
PRN	pro re nata (when required)
QDS	quater die sumendum (to be taken four times daily)
QQH	quarta quaque hora (every four hours)
SC	subcutaneous
stat	immediately
TDS	ter die sumendum (to be taken three times daily)

A further list of terms and abbreviations relevant to urgent and OOH care can be found in the Glossary (click on the Resources tab on the page for this book on the Scion website, www.scionpublishing.com)

Chapter 1: **Medico-legal aspects of providing out-of-hours medical care**

"Live your life as if your every act was to become a universal law."
Immanuel Kant

The evidence

- From 2014 to 2017 the Medical Defence Union (MDU) paid out over £30 million in compensation and legal costs for out-of-hours (evening and weekend) consultations and encounters.
- This is more than would be expected when compared to in-hours consultations; for this reason most indemnity providers will charge higher premiums for clinicians providing urgent or out-of-hours (OOH) medical care.
- In 2019/20 NHS Resolution, which manages claims for compensation on behalf of the NHS, paid out £2.3 billion in compensation[1].
- In 2019 the NHS agreed to provide limited indemnity cover to all primary care doctors working within the UK. As a result there was a significant drop in subscription charges and premiums.
- However, there is little doubt the cost of claims continues to rise.
- Several risk factors in an OOH or urgent care setting increase the risk of litigation; these include[2]:
  - diagnostic uncertainty
  - patients being more acutely unwell and the increased severity of illness
  - lack of patient medical records and unfamiliarity with the patient
  - lack of continuity of care, hence only a snapshot is obtained
  - greater use of non-face-to-face consultations, e.g. telephone
  - use of non-medically qualified staff such as call handlers and case advisors.

In 2017 the MDU provided a list of the most common causes of litigation resulting in settled claims[3]:

1. Delayed or failed diagnosis	= 71%
2. Failure to refer	= 18%
3. Medication issues	= 9%
4. Inadequate or inappropriate treatment	= 1%
5. Other	= 1%

The most common conditions which were missed or diagnosed with a delay were[3]:

1. Cauda equina syndrome
2. Limb ischaemia
3. Gastrointestinal and urological complaints: perforation, obstruction, abscess, appendicitis, testicular torsion

4. Myocardial infarction
5. Meningitis and septicaemia (in a review of 15 cases, 40% were in an OOH setting).

How to minimise the risk of complaints and litigation

- Firstly being aware of the common pitfalls helps, as well as bearing in mind that patients who present in an urgent care or OOH setting are more likely to be acutely unwell.
- When assessing a patient, key factors to consider are:
  - what is the worst-case scenario this could be? For example, if a patient presents with a headache, have I ruled out features of meningitis and documented my negative findings?
  - could the patient's condition deteriorate? If so, have I expressed my concerns to the patient and documented this in the notes?
  - note-keeping is extremely important. Always remember, if it has not been recorded in the notes it has not been done.
- Additional tips which may help to minimise the risk of litigation are:
  - review of any: past notes, previous consultations, special notes recorded on the system, summary care records or patient medical records available for sharing between healthcare organisations.
  - contemporaneous note-keeping: use quotation marks to record any key phrases the patient may use, and record negative findings, such as the absence of a rash.
  - structure to note-keeping: the mnemonic SOAPS can be used as a framework:
    Subjective findings: e.g. patient looked well, alert, smiling, and comfortable
    Objective findings: e.g. pulse, temperature, BP, blood glucose, SpO_2
    Assessment: what you think the diagnosis is, e.g. viral infection
    Plan: what the plan is, e.g. advised rest, paracetamol, fluids
    Safety-net: advise the patient of worsening features to look out for and what to do if they occur; document this advice.
  - amending records: always record the date and time the records were amended.
- Building a rapport with your patients is key. What you do not want to do is leave gunpowder all over the place; all it takes is for something to go wrong – i.e. a spark – and then we have an explosion, i.e. a complaint or litigation. Patients are less likely to complain about a doctor they like, even when that doctor gets it wrong.
- Key tips on building a rapport:
  - ICE: elicit ideas and concerns and manage those expectations. Key phrases can help in achieving this, e.g. *'What were your thoughts?'*, *'Was there anything you were concerned about?'*, *'What are your thoughts as to where we go from here?'*, *'What were you hoping I could do for you today?'*
  - Perceived arrogance, rudeness or inattention can lead to a complaint.
  - Arrange a follow-up if necessary with the patient's own GP by sending an email or electronic post-event message (PEM). Most organisations will send a PEM to the patient's practice; mention this to the patient, although it may take 48–72 hours for the practice to receive it. Give the patient a referral letter if an onward referral to secondary care is needed.

Safety-netting and additional points to remember

- The importance of safety-netting cannot be stressed enough, especially when there is diagnostic uncertainty.
- Safety-netting plays an essential role in minimising the risk of complications and the likelihood of the patient deteriorating.
- When there is diagnostic uncertainty consider calling a colleague in for a second opinion; document that the patient was seen with Dr X or Nurse Y and what the agreed diagnosis and management plan was.
- If performing an intimate examination always offer a chaperone; this should be someone who is the same gender as the patient.
- Document the presence of a chaperone (use their initials or first name) or the patient's refusal to have a chaperone, in your contemporaneous notes.
- Always try to record a diagnosis or impression in the records.
- Follow local or national guidance on management of common conditions; guidelines should be available on the local intranet or internet.
- Specify a timeframe in which you expect the patient to become better or recover.
- If the patient is not well after this advise them to seek medical attention; record this in the notes.
- Always safety-net and record any advice in your notes; e.g. 'advised if no better in 72 hours / worse / concerns call back, or own GP'.
- Appropriate safety-netting and documentation of safety-netting carries more weight in a court of law than recording your clinical findings.
- Mention complications which could arise, and be specific, e.g. vomiting post head injuries. Document that you have discussed the possibility of complications with the patient and advised them to seek medical attention should they occur. Often I will advise the patient or carer if they have any concerns to seek medical attention, and document this advice.
- Offer patient information leaflets if available or printouts from patient information websites such as www.patient.co.uk and www.nhs.uk.
- Document that you gave the patient an information leaflet.
- Check the patient's understanding using direct questioning; e.g. *'just to make sure I have explained everything correctly I'd be grateful if you could tell me exactly what complications you should look out for and what to do if they occur'*.
- If necessary, and with the patient's consent, call a family member or a friend of the patient into the room and discuss your findings and plan with them.
- Record the names of everyone present in the room during your consultation.
- It is essential to remember that even when a healthcare professional conducts a thorough assessment and implements an appropriate management plan, patients can still become unwell.
- It is vital that clinical notes are contemporaneous and reflect an accurate and objective assessment of the patient.
- In a court of law the clinician will be required to justify their actions based on the clinical notes and any recollection of events during the consultation.
- The importance of safety-netting and documentation of this advice cannot be stressed enough.

Summary for medico-legal aspects of providing OOH care

- The most common reasons for litigation are: delayed or failed diagnosis, failure to refer, medication issues, and inadequate or inappropriate treatment.
- The most common conditions that were missed or diagnosed with a delay were: cauda equina syndrome, limb ischaemia, gastrointestinal and urological complaints, myocardial infarction, meningitis and septicaemia.
- Minimise this risk of a missed diagnosis by:
    - reviewing past or special notes, utilising structured consultations and conducting a thorough examination
    - considering a second opinion from a colleague
    - ensuring accurate and detailed record-keeping.
- Build a rapport with your patient.
- Use the mnemonic SOAPS to structure note-keeping.
- Safety-net and document your advice and arrange a follow-up if necessary.

References

1. NHS Resolution (2020) *Annual report and accounts 2019/20*. Available at: https://resolution.nhs.uk/2020/07/16/nhs-resolutions-annual-report-and-accounts-2019-20

2. MDU (2018) *Urgent action needed to curb compensation payouts.*

3. MDU (2017) *Why are unscheduled or out of hours consultations more risky?*

Chapter 2: **Telephone consultations and telephone triage**

"Emails get reactions, phone calls start conversations."
Simon Sinek

Remember the risks

- Telephone consultations carry with them an inherent risk, primarily because the clinician cannot assess the patient face-to-face and conduct a physical examination.
- In addition any non-verbal cues are missed and it may be difficult to ascertain the exact nature of the problem.
- Nonetheless, telephone consultations play an essential role in providing urgent medical care both in and out of hours, and in some cases patients prefer them.

History-taking

- It is essential to confirm the identity of the patient, and at least three patient-specific details should be confirmed prior to beginning the consultation. These can be their name, date of birth, address or telephone number.
- When consulting via telephone it is good practice to start with an introduction, mention your name and also the organisation you are calling on behalf of; an example would be '*Good morning, this is Dr X and I am calling from the out-of-hours GP service*'.
- If a relative or friend is calling on behalf of the patient, ask if you can talk to the patient.
- Ask if there is anyone else in the room and confirm their names and relationship to the patient.
- Start with open questions such as *'What can I help you with today?'*
- Then move to closed questions and ask about 'red flag' features, e.g. '*Are you having any bowel or bladder problems with your back pain?*'
- Ask questions about previous occurrences or similar symptoms and how they were managed.
- Enquire about a medical, surgical, psychiatric, immunisation and social history.
- Ask about any medications the patient may be on and whether they have any allergies.
- Occasionally a patient will state that they do not have any medical problems but then provide a list of several medications they may be taking.
- Enquire about any recent travel abroad.
- If available ask for permission to access the patient's SCR (summary care record) or PMR (patient medical record).
- If there is someone else in the room, and talking to them would assist in gathering further information, do so with the consent of the patient.

- Try to elicit the patient's ideas, concerns and the reason for the call along with expectations.
- Summarise the history the patient has given you; this is a good way to show active listening skills and also to ensure the history obtained is correct.

Conducting an assessment

- The patient may have diagnostic equipment at home such as a thermometer, pulse oximeter, sphygmomanometer, blood glucose meter or peak flow meter.
- Enquire about diagnostic equipment and if they have been used, and what the readings are.
- Even without diagnostic aids the patient may also be able to provide basic observations such as the pulse rate and respiratory rate; they may also be able to palpate for tenderness over the affected area.
- If there is a healthcare professional in the room, ask if they are able to use any diagnostic equipment to obtain observations which may assist in confirming the diagnosis.
- Document these findings in your contemporaneous notes.
- Assess the patient's speech on the phone:
  - does the patient sound comfortable?
  - is the patient talking in complete sentences?
  - is the patient coherent?
  - is the patient distressed and in pain?
- Document your assessment in your contemporaneous notes.

Agree a shared management plan

- Tell the patient what you think may be wrong or what the diagnosis could be; reassure the patient if their concerns are unfounded.
- Avoid medical terminology and empathise with the patient.
- Determine expectations: not all patients will want a visit or face-to-face consultation; some may just want advice.
- Have a low threshold for booking face-to-face consultations for children and the elderly.
- If the patient has had two or more remote consultations and the problem has not been resolved, consider a face-to-face assessment.
- Try to manage expectations: for example, OOH primary care services may not have access to imaging or controlled drugs, and it is important to let patients know this.

Managing difficult consultations

- Apologise for any delays:
  - *'I am sorry you had to wait so long for a call back'*
- Show empathy and acknowledge the patient's feelings.
  - *'I understand... I get the feeling... I sense you are angry...'*
- Defuse any hostility by using the 'I agree' statement:
  - *'I agree with you that this is most likely the flu, caused by a virus; however, antibiotics will not help'*
  - *'I agree this is not an ideal situation'*
- If the consultation is unsalvageable offer a second contact with a colleague.

- Ideally all telephone consultations should be recorded and most OOH provider organisations will and should have processes in place to ensure this.
- Avoid using your own mobile phone.
- Contemporaneous note-keeping is essential.

Remote prescribing

- On some occasions the diagnosis will be clear on the phone and the patient will require a prescription for medication.
- Often the patient may be presenting with a recurrence of a problem that was treated in the past with a course of medication.
- Most OOH providers now have software in place where a prescription can be sent electronically to a pharmacy and the patient or the next of kin is then able to pick up the medication.
- If you are going to issue a prescription remotely, ensure the patient details are correct and the patient or next of kin is aware which pharmacy to go to and how long it will be before the medication is ready to be picked up.
- Ensure there is a clear record in the patient's notes of the duration and quantity of medication prescribed, along with any instructions.
- Issue a full course of medication for any specific conditions, e.g. 7 days of antibiotics for a complicated urinary tract infection.
- Pharmacists can issue an emergency supply of repeat medication (visible on the patient's medical or summary care records) at their discretion and without the need for a prescription; however, the patient may have to pay for the medication, even if they are normally exempt from prescription charges.
- Avoid issuing prescriptions for controlled drugs unless it is absolutely necessary, e.g. palliative care patients who require immediate pain relief.
- Only issue enough repeat medication until the patient is able to see their own GP.
- Beware of repeat callers who are seeking controlled drugs; if this is suspected then raise your suspicions with the clinical lead or medical director of the OOH organisation.
- If there is any doubt regarding the issuing of a remote prescription, consider a face-to-face assessment.

Outcomes

- Based on your telephone consultation the following outcomes may be reached; in each case it is important to remember key factors.

1. Advice:

- Agree a plan of action or management.
- A remote or electronic prescription sent to the patient's pharmacy of choice.
- Safety-net, e.g. *'If symptoms worsen or are no better in 4–6 hours please call back.'*
- Ensure the patient has understood the plan and safety-netting advice and is happy with it.
- Occasionally you may opt for a second contact in a few hours in order to reassess the patient after providing telephone advice. Reaffirm this by letting the patient know that you or your colleague will call back within a specified timeframe.

2. Face-to-face consultation:
- Agree the date, time and venue of the consultation.
- Give directions to the clinic if these are required.
- Some organisations will expect the clinician to book the patient in for an appointment; others may have a dedicated call centre, in which case advise the patient that they should receive a call in the next few minutes indicating the location and time of the face-to-face consultation.
- Safety-net, advising if symptoms worsen then the patient should call back to make the clinician and OOH service aware so a further assessment can be conducted.

3. Home visit:
- These are usually reserved for bed- or housebound patients; have all patient information at hand including clinical observations.
- Advise timeframes – these can vary depending on resources available and demand.
- Safety-net, advising the patient that if symptoms worsen they should call back.

4. Ambulance:
- The clinician should make the call to the ambulance control room.
- Document the time of the call and the reference number given by ambulance control.
- Phone the patient and inform them that you have requested an ambulance.
- As of 2021 changes in NHS software now allow an ambulance to be dispatched using an online module which can be built into the note-keeping software.
- Advise on timeframes and advise that if an ambulance has not arrived within a specified timeframe, to call back.
- The different categories of ambulance dispositions and their target response times (for 90% of calls) are listed below:
  - category 1 ambulance – this is for life-threatening conditions such as cardiac and respiratory arrest; the response time is 15 minutes
  - category 2 ambulance – this is for serious conditions such as a stroke which requires a rapid assessment and transport; the response time is 40 minutes
  - category 3 ambulance – this is for urgent problems such as non-severe burns and early stages of labour; the response time is 2 hours
  - category 4 ambulance – this is for non-urgent conditions and where a transfer to hospital is required; the response time is 3 hours.
- Ensure a relative or friend stays with the patient whilst an ambulance is on the way; occasionally it may be necessary for a clinician to stay with the patient until an ambulance arrives.
- Advise the patient to call back or dial 999 if the symptoms become worse.

5. You may also refer the patient to other local services:
- Online resources, e.g. www.nhs.uk
- Dentist
- Pharmacy (consider referring the patient to the Pharmacy First Scheme[1] (available in England); this is where pharmacists are trained to assess and treat specific conditions such as acute otitis media, impetigo and sore throats)
- Social services
- Mental health services

- District nurses
- Emergency Department (ED)
- Urgent Treatment Centre (UTC)
- Urgent Care Centre (UCC)
- Minor Injuries and Illness Unit (MIIU).

Summary for telephone consultations and telephone triage

- Remember that remote consultations carry more risk.
- Identify the patient and introduce yourself.
- The patient may have some diagnostic equipment present which can aid in determining the diagnosis.
- Have a low threshold for booking face-to-face consultations for children and the elderly.
- Manage expectations.

Reference

1. NHS England (undated) *Pharmacy First*. Available at: www.england.nhs.uk/primary-care/pharmacy/pharmacy-services/pharmacy-first

3

Chapter 3: **Video consultations**

"The day will come when the man at the telephone will be able to see the distant person to whom he is speaking."
Alexander Graham Bell

Setting the scene

- The coronavirus pandemic which began in 2020 has resulted in a large number of consultations being done remotely, and video consultations are increasing in popularity.
- They allow visual information and clues to be obtained immediately, something which cannot be done via telephone consultations.
- As with telephone consultations it is important to confirm the patient's identity.
- As the patient will be able to see you, it is important to dress appropriately.
- It is vital to look at the camera and not the screen, otherwise the patient may get the impression you are not fully engaged.
- This can be difficult and one way around this is to ensure the camera is as close to the screen as possible.
- Ensure any lighting source is behind the camera and not behind you.
- Avoid distractions, as the patient will feel you are not paying attention.

Assessing the patient via video consultation

- Once the identity of the patient or caller has been confirmed, introduce yourself.
- Confirm the names and relationships of any other people in the room.
- The quality of the video and audio will very much depend on the internet connection and equipment available, hence you can ask for still images to be emailed or sent via add-on messaging software such as AccuRx.
- A video consultation will allow you to pick up visual signs such as respiratory rate, pallor and cyanosis. You can also ask the patient to measure their pulse rate and place their hand on their chest to determine the depth and rate of respiration.
- A patient who is still in bed in the afternoon is more likely to be unwell, compared to someone who has taken the time and effort to get out of bed and get dressed.
- If it is difficult to see the patient, ask them to move into the light or to ensure any lighting source or a window is behind the camera.
- Additional lighting can be used to assess parts of the body, e.g. a torch to assess for tonsillitis.
- If the patient has any diagnostic equipment at home, ask them to use it and obtain some observations; these will assist in ascertaining the diagnosis.
- The patient will also be able to point to the affected areas of the body as well as to palpate for tenderness and masses.
- Skin lesions can be assessed using still or video images along with a ruler or an object such as a coin to determine their size and distance from anatomical landmarks.
- Rashes can also be assessed to see if they are blanching or non-blanching using the glass test.

- Range of movement of the joints and the musculoskeletal system can also be assessed, as well as any deformities, swellings and wounds.

Glass test

This is used to determine if a rash is blanching or non-blanching. If the rash can be seen through a glass tumbler when it is pressed on the skin, it is considered to be non-blanching.

Outcomes

- Although video consultations are an excellent way of assessing patients remotely, one must not hesitate to opt for a face-to-face consultation, especially if there are any doubts or concerns with regard to the aetiology of the patient's problem.
- Come to a shared management plan.
- If the diagnosis is clear and medication is required, then a prescription can be issued remotely or electronically.
- Ensure appropriate safety-netting.
- Once again have a low threshold for children and the elderly with regard to booking face-to-face consultations.
- If the patient has had two or more remote consultations and the problem has not been resolved, consider a face-to-face assessment.

Summary for video consultations

- Remember that remote consultations carry more risk.
- Identify the patient and introduce yourself.
- When compared to telephone consultations, video consultations allow for additional information to be obtained.
- The patient will be able to point to the affected area and palpate for tenderness.
- Consider additional lighting.
- Video quality will depend on the equipment used.
- Have a low threshold for booking face-to-face consultations for children and the elderly.

4

Chapter 4: **Home visits**

"The good physician treats the disease, the great physician treats the person who has the disease."
William Osler

Before setting off

- Home visits are a valuable resource and generally a home visit will take longer to complete than a clinic consultation, as the time taken to conduct a home visit will include travelling to and from the patient's home.
- There are limitations to what can be achieved on home visits, especially when compared to seeing a patient in a clinic setting. There may be limited space, equipment and colleague support available.
- OOH organisations will provide a car, driver, telephone and a computer to record clinical notes.
- Most cars will be equipped with a nebuliser, defibrillator, medication, controlled drugs and consumables such as gloves and syringes.
- Personal protective equipment (PPE) should also be readily available.
- It is important to familiarise yourself with what is available and where it is kept in the car.
- It will be necessary to prioritise visits according to clinical need. Prior to setting off, give the patient an estimated timeframe within which you intend to arrive, and advise the patient to call back if symptoms worsen.
- Occasionally you may have to call the patient whilst in the car, to reassess whether their condition has changed and whether an ambulance is required, or whether the patient can continue to wait for a home visit.
- Always wear an identity badge with a photograph; this should be worn where it can be seen by patients and their relatives.

Assessing a patient on a home visit

- On arrival it is important to ensure it is safe to enter the premises. Always be wary of pets, especially those that can bite – the last thing you want is to end up at the local Emergency Department (ED) as a patient.
- Introduce yourself and the organisation you are representing.
- Confirm who the patient is and the names of any friends or relatives who are present during the consultation, and record these in your notes.
- A good bedside manner is important.
- Try not to lean over the patient; stay at eye level.
- Talk in a calm, coherent manner and empathise with the patient.
- Try to keep contemporaneous notes.
- Some OOH organisations will provide you with a portable device such as a laptop or tablet; you can take this into the patient's home with you, or keep handwritten notes which you can then transfer onto the computer in the car.

- Ensure any paper notes which contain confidential patient data are disposed of appropriately.
- Record your consultation and examination findings.
- Using the mnemonic SOAPS to structure your notes will help.

Management plan and issuing a prescription

- Put a shared management plan in place and try to meet the patient's expectations.
- If you are dispensing medication from the medicine stock in the car, record the name of the medication and the quantity dispensed.
- Record the batch number and expiry date of any dispensed medication.
- Some organisations will request that this be recorded on the dispensing module of the record-keeping software; alternatively it can be free-texted into your notes.
- If issuing an FP10 prescription, ensure you write clearly and include all patient details. It is good practice to write in capital letters and specify exact instructions.
- To avoid ambiguity, spell out any numbers in brackets.
- Cross through any part of the prescription that is not used. Record your name and your prescriber or regulatory body number next to your signature.
- A log should be kept of every FP10 prescription issued – this should include the name of the clinician who has issued it and the case number or patient it applies to.
- Safety-net and let the patient know in what timeframe you expect them to get better and if this does not occur, then to seek medical advice.

Referring a patient to hospital

- If the patient requires an onward referral to hospital, use the telephone provided by the OOH organisation to make any calls.
- Ensure you document the time you spoke to the person accepting the referral and also their name.
- Be clear about whether you are requesting a clinical assessment for your patient or are asking for advice.
- Provide the patient with a letter and also ensure there is adequate transportation.
- In some cases a patient may prefer to have a relative or friend take them by car to the nearest hospital rather than an ambulance; always document this.
- If you are arranging an ambulance, then most OOH organisations will have a direct number to the ambulance service.
- Life-threatening or medical emergencies should have an emergency ambulance (category 1 or 2) arranged.
- It is good practice to wait with the patient whilst an emergency ambulance arrives, as a good verbal handover to the ambulance crew is important. Also provide a letter which the ambulance crew can hand over to the doctors in hospital.
- For routine transfers a 1–4-hour ambulance may be sufficient; provided there is someone with the patient, you do not have to wait for the ambulance.
- Inform the patient and relative of the estimated time of arrival of the ambulance and advise that if symptoms worsen, they should call back or dial 999.
- The ambulance service will provide you with a reference number and this can be given to the patient or carer to use if a repeat call to the ambulance service is required.

Summary for home visits

- Home visits take more time and there are limitations to what can be achieved.
- Ensure you have the right equipment, including a manual sphygmomanometer.
- When assessing a patient be empathetic and remain at eye level.
- Safety-net.
- Consider waiting with the patient for an emergency ambulance.

5

Chapter 5: **Head injuries**

"One day we will learn that the heart can never be totally right if the head is totally wrong. Only through the bringing together of head and heart – intelligence and goodness – shall man rise to a fulfilment of his true nature."

Martin Luther King, Jr

Acute presentations of head injuries are relatively uncommon in primary care as most patients with acute head injuries will be assessed in the ED or in an Urgent Treatment Centre (UTC).

On the odd occasion you may see a patient in primary care, it may be because the patient may have developed symptoms a few days after the initial injury, or may require reassurance that the vague symptoms they are experiencing are not due to a serious complication as a result of the head injury.

Assessment of patients presenting with head injuries

Telephone

- A detailed history can be taken over the phone.
- Always ask about head trauma in anyone who has had a fall, especially the elderly.
- Red flag features such as limb or facial weakness can be queried over the phone.
- The presence of any open wounds or deformities should also be queried.
- On some occasions a direct referral to ED may be required and in such cases, ambulance transfer should be considered.

Face-to-face

This is required if the history is unclear, there is a possibility of complications or the patient requires reassurance via a physical examination.

Face-to-face assessment of patients with head injuries

- A full assessment should consist of checking the pulse, blood pressure, oxygen saturations, temperature and capillary glucose levels.
- A full peripheral neurological examination including power, tone and reflexes of all limbs should be undertaken.
- Features suggestive of a cerebellar injury are a positive Romberg's test, past pointing, dysdiadochokinesis (impaired ability to perform rapidly alternating movements), nystagmus and staccato speech.
- Examine all the cranial nerves (CN):

- olfactory (CN I) – ask the patient about their sense of smell
- ophthalmic (CN II) – check reaction of pupils to light and accommodation
- oculomotor (CN III), trochlear (CN IV), abducens (CN VI) – check eye movements
- trigeminal (CN V)
  - sensory division (ophthalmic, maxillary, mandibular branches) – check sensation
  - motor division – ask patient to open the mouth against resistance and to clench the jaw
- facial (CN VII) – check facial movements
- vestibulocochlear (CN VIII) – check hearing
- glossopharyngeal (CN IX), vagus (CN X) – ask the patient to open their mouth and say 'aah'; look for appropriate elevation of the pharynx
- accessory (CN XI) – check shoulder and neck movements
- hypoglossal (CN XII) – check tongue movements.

The Glasgow Coma Scale (GCS) can be used to quantify any impairment in consciousness[1]:

	1	2	3	4	5	6
Eye	Does not open eyes	Opens eyes in response to painful stimuli	Opens eyes in response to voice	Opens eyes spontaneously	N/A	N/A
Verbal	Makes no sounds	Incomprehensible sounds	Utters incoherent words	Confused, disoriented	Oriented, converses normally	N/A
Motor	Makes no movements	Extension to painful stimuli (decerebrate response)	Abnormal flexion to painful stimuli (decorticate response)	Flexion / withdrawal to painful stimuli	Localises to painful stimuli	Obeys commands

The AVPU scale is another tool which can be used to assess impaired consciousness:

Alert: patient is fully awake
Verbal: patient makes a response when you talk to them
Pain: patient makes a response to pain stimuli
Unresponsive: patient does not give any eye, voice or motor response.

The AVPU scale and GCS correspond in the following manner[2]:

Alert = 15 GCS
Voice responsive = 12 GCS
Pain responsive = 8 GCS
Unconscious / life extinct = 3 GCS

Examine the head and neck for any visible injuries and record your findings.

Red flag features in patients with head injury

Patients presenting with any of the following features after a head injury should be referred to ED for assessment and a CT head scan[3]:

Altered observations	Loss of consciousness	Focal neurological deficit
Penetrating injury	Suspected skull fracture	Seizure
High-energy trauma	Amnesia	Vomiting
Previous brain surgery	Bleeding / clotting disorders	Taking anticoagulants
Drug or alcohol intoxication	Safeguarding concerns	Change in behaviour
C-spine injuries	Panda eyes	Suspected CSF leak

GCS <13 on 3 separate occasions or GCS<15 2 hours after injury.

Periorbital ecchymosis (*Fig. 5.1*), also known as 'panda eyes', indicates a basal skull fracture. Battle's sign (*Fig. 5.2*), which presents with bruising over the mastoid process, also indicates a basilar skull fracture. Patients presenting with these features should be referred to ED.

If there is a risk of developing a complication or there are concerns, then it is appropriate to discuss these with the trauma or ED doctor on call.

Any advice obtained should be documented along with the date, time and the name of the clinicians the patient was discussed with, as well as a factual summary of any advice and the management plan.

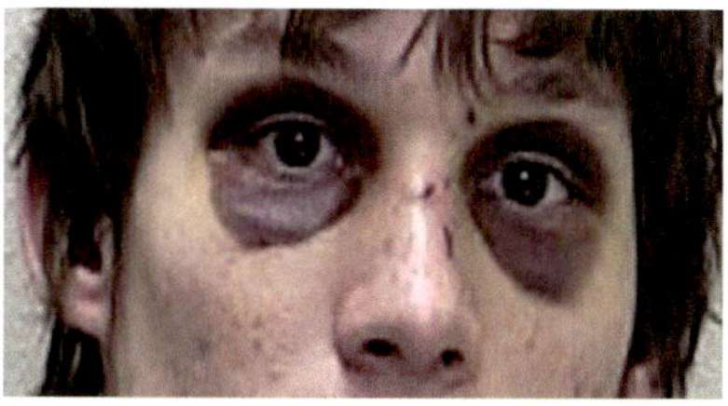

Fig. 5.1: Bilateral periorbital ecchymosis.

Reproduced from https://en.wikipedia.org/wiki/Ecchymosis#/media/File:Bilateral_periorbital_ecchymosis_(raccoon_eyes).jpg] Public domain (photo by Marion County Sheriff's Office).

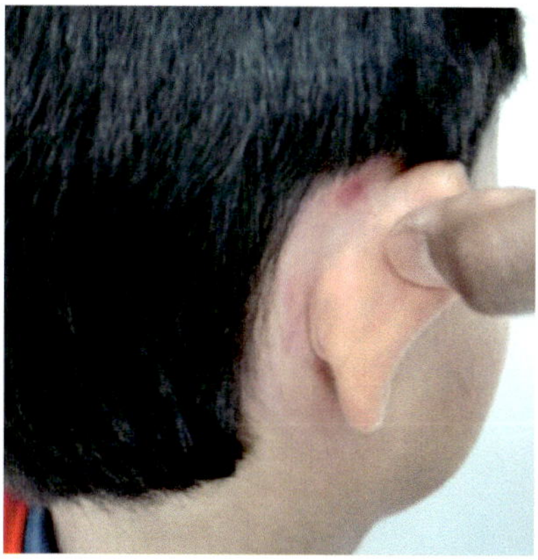

Fig. 5.2: Battle's sign – bruising over the mastoid process.

Discharging patients with minor head injuries

- The majority of patients presenting to primary care clinicians will have relatively minor head injuries and therefore will be discharged; it is important to discharge them with written and verbal advice.
- Ensure the patient will be with a responsible adult for the next 24 hours.
- Explain to the patient and carer that complications of head injuries can arise up to 48 hours later (sometimes even after 48 hours). Be specific about what to look out for, especially in children, e.g. vomiting more than twice.
- Signpost the patient or carer to where they can turn to for any future advice, such as the 111 service or the local ED.
- Mention to the patient that if they have any concerns whatsoever, to return or seek medical attention.
- Document in your contemporaneous medical notes any verbal and written advice given.

Summary for head injuries

- Take a full history and conduct a full examination.
- Remember the criteria for referral to ED and what would be considered 'red flag' features.
- Provide written advice and information leaflets.
- Safety-net and document any advice given.

References

1. Glasgow Coma Scale: www.glasgowcomascale.org/
2. Kelly, C.A., Upex, A. and Bateman, D.N. (2005) Comparison of consciousness level assessment in the poisoned patient using the alert/verbal/painful/unresponsive scale and the Glasgow Coma Scale. *Annals of Emergency Medicine*, **44**: 108–113. Available at: https://doi.org/10.1016/j.annemergmed.2004.03.028
3. NICE (updated 2019) *Head injury: assessment and early management* [CG176]. Available at: www.nice.org.uk/guidance/cg176

6

Chapter 6: **Acute injuries, bites and wounds**

Assessment of injuries, bites and wounds

Telephone

- A detailed history can be taken over the phone.
- Enquire about the location of the injury, the mechanism of injury, open wounds, active bleeding, exposed structures and any obvious deformity.
- Ask about mobility and any impact on function.
- Photographs or a video consultation can assist in determining if the patient should be referred directly to an urgent treatment centre, ED or can be managed in the community.
- Patients with minor injuries such as small abrasions can be signposted to their local pharmacist.

Face-to-face

This will be required if a bony injury is suspected, if there are open or contaminated wounds, and where it is not possible to determine the severity of the injury. Have a low threshold for the elderly and young children.

Injuries, bites and wounds

- Most injuries seen in primary care and urgent care settings tend to be soft tissue injuries, e.g. contusions, abrasions and lacerations.
- Patients who have a visible deformity of a limb or bony tenderness, or are unable to mobilise after the injury, should be referred to ED or a UTC.
- Patients with bites and wounds involving or revealing deep structures, e.g. fascia, tendons and nerves, should also be referred to ED.
- All patients should have their general observations checked; if there is an indication that blood loss is heavy then the patient should be referred to ED.
- Wounds should be cleaned thoroughly with copious amounts of saline.
- Consider X-rays to rule out bony injury or the presence of foreign bodies.
- Minor wounds can be closed using glue, steri-strips or sutures.
- Ensure the patient is up to date with their tetanus status; if not, consider administering a booster. A booster is required every 10 years unless the patient has had five tetanus injections in their lifetime.
- Antibiotic prophylaxis should be offered to all patients who have suffered an animal bite or have a contaminated wound [1].

- A typical regime is co-amoxiclav 625mg TDS or clarithromycin 500mg BD with metronidazole 400mg TDS for 7 days.
- Patients should be advised to follow up with their practice nurse or GP for a wound review in 48 hours, or sooner if complications such as infection or wound breakdown are suspected.

Reference

1. NICE (revised 2024) *Bites – human and animal. Managing a cat or dog bite*. Available at: https://cks.nice.org.uk/bites-human-and-animal#!scenario:1

7

Chapter 7: **Cardiovascular**

"I shall take the heart. For brains do not make one happy, and happiness is the best thing in the world."
The Tin Man

Assessment of patients presenting with acute cardiovascular conditions

Telephone

- In the UK the national 111 algorithms have been developed to pick up serious causes of chest pain and dyspnoea, therefore the call handler who responds to the patient's 111 call should be able to arrange an ambulance immediately. Ideally this should be done before clinical triage by a healthcare professional.
- Patients with severe chest pain of acute onset should be referred directly to ED; in such cases it is the clinician's responsibility to arrange an emergency ambulance.
- Some OOH organisations provide software that can send an instant electronic message to the ambulance service and as a result an emergency ambulance can be dispatched immediately by the triaging clinician.
- Ensure there is someone with the patient; if not, consider staying on the phone with the patient until the paramedics arrive.
- Always ask about associated symptoms such as shortness of breath, vomiting, sweating and palpitations, as these are suggestive of a serious underlying cause.
- In most cases the cause of the chest pain can be determined by taking a detailed history; serious causes should be recognised over the phone.
- Sudden onset of calf pain and swelling in those with risk factors for a DVT should warrant a face-to-face assessment or a referral to ED.

Face-to-face

This may be required in the following circumstances:

- The diagnosis is unclear, and the cause of the chest pain is not suspected to be life-threatening.
- Subacute or chronic chest pain.
- Chest pain is an associated symptom and not the dominant symptom.
- The patient requires further investigations, e.g. an ECG to rule out a cardiac cause.

Thoracic conditions causing chest pain will commonly be associated with dyspnoea, and thoracic conditions causing dyspnoea will commonly be associated with chest pain.

The causes of chest pain originating from thoracic structures can be divided into cardiac, pulmonary, gastrointestinal and muscular causes.

Abdominal aortic aneurysm (rupture)

Presentation

- This is a life-threatening emergency.
- Presentation in a primary care setting is rare, as patients will usually be transferred to hospital immediately.
- The abdominal pain will be severe and described as tearing in nature.
- On rare occasions and prior to the onset of rupture, the patient may complain of a dull ache or vague abdominal or back pain. In such cases a high index of suspicion is required.

Assessment

- Beware of the old man who presents with sudden onset of back pain; palpate for a pulsatile and expansible abdominal mass (indicative of an AAA).
- Once rupture has occurred, the patient will be unresponsive and in hypovolaemic shock.
- The abdominal cavity will be distended due to the presence of blood.
- There may be a bluish discolouration around the flanks and umbilicus, indicative of blood in the abdominal cavity.

Management

- Immediate resuscitation with intravenous fluids and emergency transfer to hospital.

Acute coronary syndrome

Presentation

- The typical presentation of ACS is of crushing central chest pain, radiating to the left jaw and down the left arm. It will be of sudden onset, lasting longer than 15 minutes.
- Common associations will be pallor, dyspnoea, diaphoresis, nausea and vomiting.
- There may be a history of predisposing factors, such as smoking, a family history of ischaemic heart disease, hypercholesterolaemia, diabetes mellitus and hypertension.

Patients who are suspected of having ACS on telephone triage should have an emergency ambulance transfer to hospital.

Assessment

- The patient will look unwell, with pallor and diaphoresis, and will be in pain.
- There may be associated tachycardia, tachypnoea, hypotension and hypoxaemia.
- Perform an ECG if available, although if there is a high index of suspicion, a negative ECG cannot be relied upon to rule out cardiac ischaemia.

Management [1], [2]

- Do not routinely administer oxygen (except for specific situations*)
- Administer morphine 5–10mg IM, cyclizine 50mg IM, aspirin 300mg PO, clopidogrel 300mg PO, GTN spray under the tongue, call 999.

- Speak to the medical team on call and arrange a time-critical transfer to the nearest ED or Coronary Care Unit (CCU).
- Always have a low index of suspicion of ACS; one can easily be caught out.
- A missed or delayed diagnosis of a myocardial infarction is one of the most common reasons for litigation.
- Sometimes patients can look relatively well and may not have typical ACS features; often various pieces of the jigsaw need to come together to confirm the diagnosis.
- If in doubt speak to the medical team on call or the senior doctor in ED.

***Only offer supplemental oxygen to the following groups:**

- Patients with SpO_2 of <94% and who are not at risk of hypercapnic respiratory failure – administer oxygen via a simple face mask at 5–10L/min aiming for SpO_2 of >94%.
- Patients who are at risk of hypercapnic respiratory failure (e.g. COPD) – administer oxygen via a 28% venturi mask at a flow rate of 4L/min aiming for SpO_2 of 88–92%.

Atypical (silent) myocardial infarctions

Presentation

- Atypical myocardial infarctions present with vague symptoms and often can be asymptomatic.
- The central crushing chest pain associated with acute coronary syndrome will be absent.
- They are more common in the elderly (>75 years of age), women and people who have diabetes mellitus.
- Presenting features include: collapse, change in sensation in the body, generalised weakness, dyspnoea, a sense of anxiety or panic, nausea or vomiting, cyanosis and palpitations.
- A high index of suspicion is required in order to diagnose a silent myocardial infarction.

A face-to-face assessment should be conducted in patients who are at risk of silent myocardial infarctions and present with vague chest or epigastric symptoms, or the presenting features listed above.

Assessment

- Observations may be within normal range and the patient may well be asymptomatic.
- ECG changes will raise the suspicion of an atypical myocardial infarction (*Fig. 7.1*), and for this reason an ECG should be considered for patients who present with the above symptoms.
- A raised serum troponin level will confirm the diagnosis.

Management

- Administer oxygen (based on the aforementioned criteria), morphine 5–10mg IM, cyclizine 50mg IM, aspirin 300mg PO, clopidogrel 300mg PO, GTN spray under the tongue, call 999.
- Speak to the medical team on call and arrange a time-critical transfer to the nearest ED or CCU.

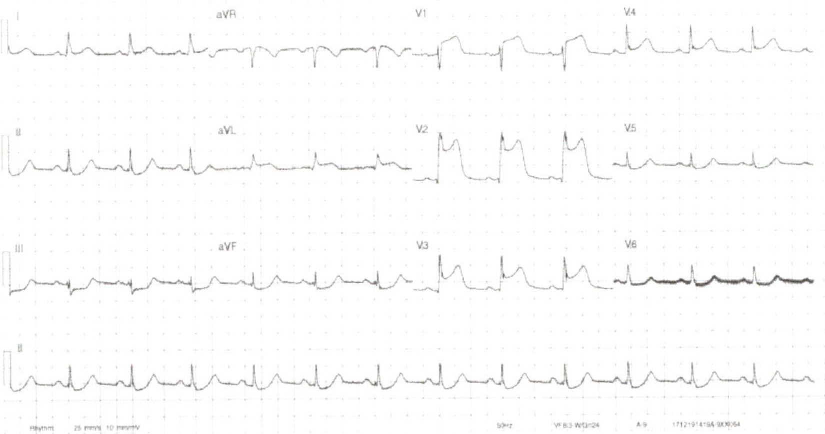

Fig. 7.1: ECG showing anterior ST segment elevation, indicative of an MI.

A missed or delayed diagnosis of a myocardial infarction is one of the most common reasons for litigation.

Stable angina

Presentation

- Stable angina refers to chest pain due to cardiac ischaemia occurring on exertion.
- Patients are pain-free at rest.
- Exertion will bring about the typical features of central chest tightness and radiation to the left arm or left jaw, along with associated symptoms such as nausea and dyspnoea.
- Symptoms will be relieved by rest.
- If there is a high index of suspicion patients should be referred directly to the Rapid Access Chest Pain Clinic (RACPC). These clinics have been set up at local hospitals to assess patients with suspected stable angina within 1 or 2 weeks.

A face-to-face assessment may help in ruling out other potential cardiac causes of exercise-induced chest pain, two examples being subacute endocarditis or aortic stenosis exercise-induced chest pain.

Assessment
- Clinical examination at rest will be entirely normal.

Management
- If stable angina is suspected start aspirin 75mg daily, prescribe GTN spray and refer the patient to the RACPC.
- Always safety-net and advise the patient that they should hear from the clinic within the next 2 weeks (waiting times vary by area).
- In the meantime if the patient has chest pain and it is severe or not relieved by GTN spray, then they must call 999.
- Always document this advice in the patient's medical records.
- Patients with unstable angina (i.e. angina occurring at rest) or with crescendo angina (angina occurring with diminishing activity) should be referred to ED or the medical team on call on the same day of presentation.

Aortic dissection

Presentation
- This occurs when the inner lining of the aorta is torn.
- It is a rare condition, occurring more often in men than women. It can occur in the thoracic or abdominal portion of the aorta.
- Patients will present with severe chest or abdominal pain.
- Often this is described as tearing in nature and radiating to the back.
- There may be precipitating factors such as a history of an aortic aneurysm, high blood pressure, trauma, bicuspid aortic valve, cocaine or amphetamine abuse, previous aortic or cardiac surgery and vascular disease.

If aortic dissection is suspected on telephone triage, an emergency ambulance should be arranged immediately.

Assessment
- There will be associated tachycardia, hypotension, tachypnoea and possible collapse.
- The lack of blood supply to distal organs may result in limb ischaemia, a stroke, mesenteric ischaemia and end organ damage.

Management
- This is a medical emergency – if you are with the patient, initiate resuscitation and refer the patient via emergency ambulance to hospital.

Pericarditis, myocarditis and endocarditis

Presentation

- These conditions refer to inflammation of the pericardium (pericarditis), myocardium (myocarditis) and endocardium (endocarditis).
- Often these conditions can be underdiagnosed or missed and require a high index of suspicion.
- The patient may initially present with fatigue only, so auscultation of the precordium in patients presenting with tiredness or fatigue is warranted in order to determine the presence of a cardiac murmur, which is indicative of endocarditis.
- There may be predisposing factors such as valvular heart disease, previous heart valve surgery, poor dentition, intravenous drug abuse, connective tissue disorders or autoimmune disorders.
- Common causes include microorganisms (viruses, bacteria, fungi), medicines (penicillin, sulphonamides), radiation, chemicals and autoimmune conditions such as granulomatosis with polyangiitis (formerly known as Wegener's granulomatosis).

Often a physical examination will be required, firstly to identify any stigmata associated with endocarditis and also to auscultate the precordium and undertake an ECG.

Features of endocarditis

- Fatigue
- Breathlessness
- Pallor
- Pyrexia
- Tachycardia
- Janeway lesions
- Osler nodes
- Splinter haemorrhages
- Cardiac murmur

Assessment

- The presence of systemic symptoms such as a high temperature, fatigue and chest pain and a cardiac murmur should raise the suspicion of endocarditis and a referral to the on-call medical team should be made.
- Additional features which may be present in endocarditis include Janeway lesions, Osler nodes and splinter haemorrhages affecting the hands and nails.
- With pericarditis a cardiac murmur will be absent; however, the chest pain and dyspnoea may be more marked. ECG changes will be present, including concave ST elevation and PR depression (see *Fig. 7.2*).
- The most common feature of myocarditis is chest pain; there will be associated pyrexia and dyspnoea. ECG changes include ST elevation, bradycardia or tachycardia and atrioventricular arrhythmias.

Management

- Patients with suspected endocarditis, myocarditis or pericarditis should be referred to the on-call medical team to confirm the diagnosis (via echocardiogram) and initiate treatment.

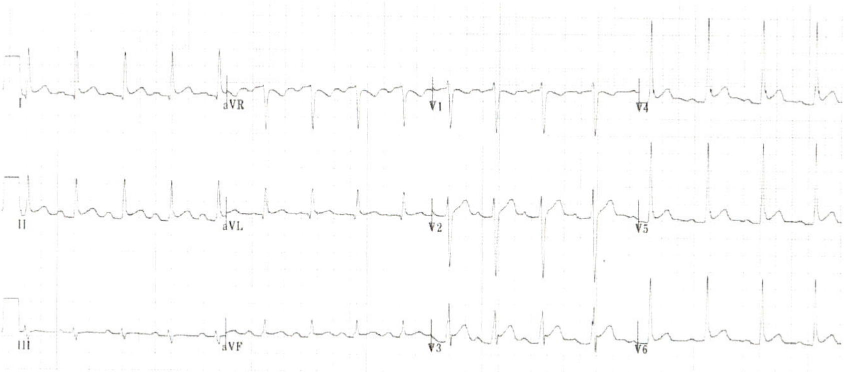

Fig. 7.2: ECG showing concave ST segment elevation and PR depression in multiple leads, indicative of pericarditis.

Reproduced from *Pericarditis*. Life in the Fast Lane: https://litfl.com/pericarditis-ecg-library/ (ECG image by Ed Burns)

Cardiac impairment (dysfunction)

Presentation

- The term 'heart failure' should be avoided; it is of very little help to the clinician and can be disheartening for patients, often implying an imminent demise.
- A more appropriate term would be cardiac impairment or dysfunction, with reference to which chambers of the heart are affected, e.g. 'left ventricular impairment' or 'biventricular impairment'.
- There may be predisposing factors such as ischaemic heart disease, hypertension, diabetes, valvular heart disease and chronic lung disease.
- Presentation will very much depend on what chambers of the heart are affected:
  - left ventricular dysfunction will present with features of pulmonary oedema such as dyspnoea, orthopnoea, paroxysmal nocturnal dyspnoea and a productive cough producing pink frothy sputum
  - right ventricular impairment will result in lower limb oedema, abdominal distension, scrotal or vulval oedema and facial oedema
  - biventricular impairment will result in a combination of the above presenting features.
- Onset of symptoms will usually be insidious.

Patients with suspected cardiac impairment will require a face-to-face assessment to determine the severity of features.

Assessment

- A general examination is essential.
- Depending on the extent, severity and the heart chambers affected, the patient may have dyspnoea, tachycardia and hypotension.
- Left ventricular impairment will result in a displaced apex beat, soft heart sounds, a 4th heart sound, weak pulses, low oxygen saturations and bibasilar coarse crepitations on auscultation of the lung fields, indicating pulmonary oedema. There may also be bibasilar dullness on percussion, indicating bilateral pleural effusions.
- Patients with right ventricular impairment may have normal observations; however, they will have features of fluid retention including facial oedema, a raised JVP, soft heart sounds, hepatomegaly, ascites, abdominal distension, scrotal or vulval oedema and lower limb oedema.
- Often in primary care the presentation will be subacute or compensated, hence the full gamut of features will not always be present.

Management

- Patients with an established diagnosis, who are stable and not in acute distress, may be managed in the community.
- A loop diuretic (e.g. furosemide) will help reduce the effects of fluid retention and alleviate symptoms. Checking the patient's weight daily can assist in assessing the effectiveness of diuresis.
- The patient should be advised to contact their own GP or cardiologist during working hours and advised that if symptoms worsen, they should seek immediate medical attention.
- Upward titration of regular medication (e.g. ACE inhibitors, beta-blockers) can be considered; however, the patient will need to be monitored.
- If the diagnosis is in doubt or the patient is acutely unwell (tachycardic, tachypnoeic, hypotensive or hypoxaemic), a referral to ED via ambulance should be arranged.

Acute limb ischaemia

Presentation

- This will affect the distal part of the limb.
- Risk factors include being elderly, trauma, clotting disorders and medication such as beta-blockers.
- Associated medical conditions predisposing patients to limb ischaemia are peripheral vascular disease, diabetes mellitus, hypertension, hypercholesterolaemia, coronary artery disease and cerebrovascular disease.
- There will be a relatively acute onset of pain and pallor or a blue hue to the affected part of the limb.
- Patients may also complain of numbness or pins and needles.

If there is a strong index of suspicion on telephone triage then consider a direct referral to ED or the on-call vascular surgeons. A video consultation may assist in assessing the colour of the limb and capillary refill time.

Assessment

- On examination the affected part of the limb will appear pale or have a bluish discolouration (*Fig. 7.3*), it will feel cold and the pulses will be absent (confirmed by Doppler ultrasound) or diminished.
- Capillary refill time will be >2 seconds.

Management

- An immediate referral to the local ED or on-call vascular surgeon is mandatory.

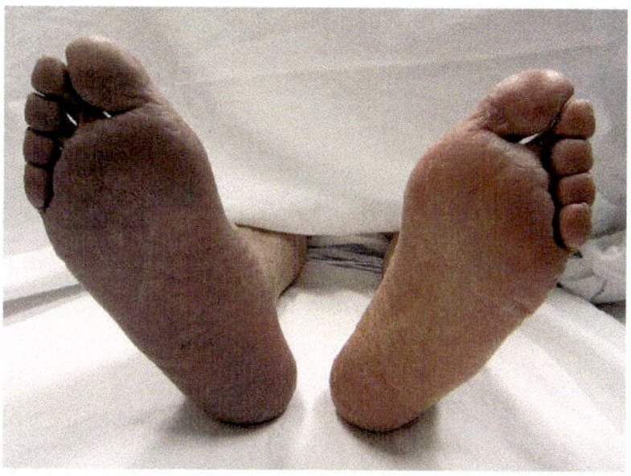

Fig. 7.3: Cyanosis of the right foot distal to an occlusion caused by acute arterial thrombosis of the right leg.

Reproduced from https://commons.wikimedia.org/wiki/File:Arterial_thrombosis_causing_cyanosis.jpg under a CC BY-SA 3.0 licence. Photo by James Heilman, MD.

Hypertensive crisis (malignant hypertension)[3]

Presentation

- Although hypertension is a chronic medical condition usually managed by the patient's own GP, hypertensive crisis can develop acutely and present with life-threatening complications.
- A hypertensive crisis is defined by a systolic blood pressure (SBP) >180mmHg and/or a diastolic blood pressure (DBP) >120mmHg.
- Causes include non-compliance with medication, renovascular disease, vasculitis, head injury and drug intoxication (e.g. amphetamines, cocaine).
- Patients may be asymptomatic and an elevated blood pressure reading may be an incidental finding.
- Although it is an acute vascular condition it can often present with neurological manifestations.
- Presenting features may include a headache, visual disturbances, epistaxis and palpitations, as well as features suggestive of acute complications.
- Patients are at risk of serious end organ damage including encephalopathy, intracerebral haemorrhage, acute heart failure, pulmonary oedema, acute kidney injury and visual loss.

A face-to-face assessment will be required if malignant hypertension or a hypertensive crisis is suspected. Some patients may have an automated blood pressure monitor at home; however, this may be inaccurate and it will not always pick up a very high or very low blood pressure reading.

Assessment

- Blood pressure readings should be taken manually and from both arms.
- Any complications should be looked for, so a full cardiovascular and respiratory examination should be undertaken.
- Fundoscopy may be required to assess for retinal haemorrhages.
- Urinalysis should be undertaken to identify the presence of protein and blood in the urine, which can be indicative of renal injury.

Management

- Patients with hypertensive crisis should be referred to ED as the blood pressure will need to be brought down in a controlled manner and IV medication (e.g. labetalol) may be required to do this.

Deep vein thrombosis

Presentation

- A deep vein thrombosis (DVT) will present with relatively sudden onset of pain in the calf.
- Risk factors include being elderly, prolonged immobilisation, underlying malignancy, clotting disorders and a previous history of DVT or pulmonary embolism (PE).

All patients with a suspected DVT should have a face-to-face assessment.

Assessment [4]

- The presenting features will be swelling (>5cm in circumference when compared to the contralateral limb), tenderness, firmness and the sudden appearance of new varicosities.
- Normal skin appearance and temperature over the affected area will assist in differentiating it from cellulitis.
- The Wells score (see below) can also be used to assess patients for a DVT [5].
- Patients with a suspected DVT should be referred to ED or an urgent treatment centre which has appropriate facilities to assess further, i.e. blood tests (D-dimer) and Doppler scans.

Two-level DVT Wells score

Clinical feature	Points	Patient score
Active cancer (treatment ongoing, within 6 months, or palliative)	1	
Paralysis, paresis or recent plaster immobilisation of the lower extremities	1	
Recently bedridden for ≥3 days or major surgery within 12 weeks requiring general or regional anaesthesia	1	
Localised tenderness along the distribution of the deep venous system	1	

Clinical feature	Points	Patient score
Entire leg swollen	1	
Calf swelling at least 3cm larger than asymptomatic side	1	
Pitting oedema confined to the symptomatic leg	1	
Collateral superficial veins (non-varicose)	1	
Previously documented DVT	1	
An alternative diagnosis is at least as likely as DVT	−2	
Clinical probability simplified score		
DVT *likely*	≥2	
DVT *unlikely*	≤1	

Bilateral lower limb oedema (ankle swelling)

Presentation

- Usually this will be of an insidious onset unless it is due to a DVT (in which case it will be unilateral and associated with pain).
- Patients may have a history of recurrent episodes managed with a diuretic.
- Common causes are obesity, pregnancy, chronic venous insufficiency, right ventricular or biventricular impairment, hypothyroidism, postural, medication (calcium channel blockers, corticosteroids, oral contraception), trauma and chronic kidney disease (nephrotic syndrome).

Often the cause will be apparent on telephone triage and patients will have been managed in the past with a diuretic. If the patient is unwell or serious underlying pathology is suspected then a face-to-face assessment should be arranged.

Assessment

- Assess and record general observations.
- Assess for signs of cardiac impairment.
- Assess for features suggestive of a DVT.
- Palpate the abdomen for ascites and to assess for any intra-abdominal masses which may be causing pressure on the inferior vena cava.
- Consider urinalysis if nephrotic syndrome is suspected.

Management

- The underlying cause should be sought and treated. Often in an urgent care setting this may not be possible and the aim of treatment will be resolution of the oedema until the patient's own GP can further investigate the causes of the oedema.
- Elevation of the limbs and a loop diuretic, e.g. furosemide 20–40mg OD for 7 days, will help to reduce the oedema.
- Daily weighing can assist in ascertaining the effectiveness of diuresis.

- The patient must be advised that if symptoms worsen or there are any concerns, medical attention should be sought.
- If the patient is acutely unwell or a potentially serious cause is suspected such as a DVT, the patient should be referred to the on-call medical team.

Syncope

Presentation

- Syncope occurs when a person's blood pressure drops, resulting in a temporary disruption of blood flow to the brain and causing a temporary loss of consciousness.
- The most common cause of syncope is vasovagal syncope, which occurs due to hyperstimulation of the vagus nerve resulting in vasodilation. It can be triggered by emotional or physical stress.
- Other causes of syncope include hypotension, arrhythmias, dehydration, hypoglycaemia, electrolyte abnormalities, pulmonary embolism, cerebrovascular accidents and seizures.
- Presenting features include pallor, blurred vision, light-headedness, nausea and sweating.
- During an episode the patient may exhibit limb jerking.
- Incontinence and tongue biting are suggestive of a seizure and not vasovagal syncope.
- Resolution is rapid and there are no residual neurological deficits.
- Often patients may have recurrent episodes.

A detailed history can be taken over the phone. The presence of an obvious trigger and absence of red flag features, such as incontinence and chest pain, support the diagnosis of vasovagal syncope.

Rapid resolution and the absence of any residual symptoms suggest vasovagal syncope; in such cases reassurance and advice can be provided via telephone.

If there are residual symptoms or features suggesting an alternative cause, a face-to-face assessment should be arranged.

Assessment

- Assess for any injuries.
- All patients should have their general observation assessed, including blood glucose levels and postural blood pressure readings (sitting and standing).
- Auscultate the precordium to determine if there are any underlying cardiac abnormalities, e.g. an ejection systolic murmur, which is a feature of aortic stenosis (a cause of exertional syncope).
- A full neurological assessment should also be undertaken to rule out any neurological deficit.
- If possible, consider performing an ECG.

Management

- Patients with suspected vasovagal syncope can be reassured and discharged back to the care of their GP.
- Address any underlying contributory factors such as dehydration or hypoglycaemia by advising the patient to maintain adequate hydration and avoid prolonged fasting.
- Advise the patient to avoid any emotional triggers which may precipitate a repeat episode.
- Patients with suspected underlying cardiology problems should be referred to the on-call cardiology team.
- If a neurological cause is suspected, the patient should be advised to speak to their own GP and to consider a referral to a neurologist.

Summary for cardiovascular

- Beware of the old man who presents with sudden onset of back pain – think AAA!
- ACS must be ruled out when assessing patients presenting with acute chest pain.
- ECGs can be normal in patients who have ACS.
- The presence of a cardiac murmur in patients presenting with fatigue or pyrexia of unknown origin should raise the suspicion of endocarditis.
- Skin conditions such as shingles can be a cause of chest pain, so always assess the skin.

References

1. NICE (revised 2022) CKS: *Chest pain – management*. Available at: https://cks.nice.org.uk/topics/chest-pain/management/management/

2. Switaj, T.L. (2017) Acute coronary syndrome: current treatment. *American Family Physician*, **95(4):** 232–240.

3. Naranjo, M. and Paul, M. (updated 2023) *Malignant hypertension*. StatPearls. Available at: www.ncbi.nlm.nih.gov/books/NBK507701/

4. NICE (revised 2023) *Deep vein thrombosis*. Available at: https://cks.nice.org.uk/deep-vein-thrombosis#!topicSummary

5. Tenna, A.S., Harrison, S., Avital, L. and Stansby, G. (2012) The two-level Wells scores should be used in suspected VTE cases. September 2012. *Guidelines in Practice*.

8

Chapter 8: Respiratory

"Breathing is the greatest pleasure in life."
Giovanni Papini

Assessment of patients presenting with acute respiratory conditions

Telephone

- Dyspnoea is not always the predominant presenting condition in patients with an acute respiratory condition; often there will be associated symptoms such as pain and cough, so it is important to enquire about these.
- It should be noted that several non-thoracic conditions, such as sepsis, can also present with shortness of breath.
- Dyspnoea is associated with severe pain and anxiety and if the presenting complaint is solely shortness of breath, one should not assume the cause is always above the diaphragm.
- A detailed history can usually be taken over the phone unless the patient is severely dyspnoeic. Often this will be obvious on the telephone and in such cases an emergency ambulance should be arranged.
- Additional sounds such as a wheeze or stridor may be heard.
- If the patient can talk in complete sentences, this is a reassuring sign.
- The ability to ascend stairs at home or walk 50 metres is another reassuring sign.
- Patients may be able to measure their own respiratory rate and describe the depth of their breaths.
- Some patients may have a pulse oximeter at home; this can be used to measure the pulse rate and oxygen saturations.
- Patients with asthma may have a peak flow meter and this can be used to gauge the severity of any bronchoconstriction.
- A video consultation can help in identifying cyanosis, recessions, shallow breathing and the respiratory rate.

Face-to-face

A face-to-face assessment will be required in the following circumstances:

- The diagnosis is unclear on the history alone.
- A further assessment is required to determine the severity of the underlying condition.
- The patient is at high risk of developing complications.
- Further investigations such as a chest X-ray may be required.
- Treatment such as a nebuliser is required.

Asthma

Presentation

- Patients will usually have a pre-existing history of asthma.
- Compliance with medication should be queried, as well as poor inhaler technique, both of which can be causes of frequent exacerbations. For these reasons it is always worth asking the patient to demonstrate their inhaler technique via video consultation or in person.
- I have come across a patient who sprayed the inhaler directly onto her chest as she thought this would 'open up her lungs quicker', so always take the time to assess technique.
- The patient will be wheezy, chesty and complain of a 'tight chest'.
- There may often be propagating factors such as poor inhaler technique, poor compliance with medication, weather changes, pollen or respiratory tract infections.

Patients who know their asthma well may already have a management plan in place and may just require a prescription for an emergency supply of medication such as oral prednisolone. These patients can usually be triaged over the phone and a prescription sent electronically to their nominated pharmacy. However, if there are doubts about the severity of the exacerbation or the underlying trigger, consider a face-to-face assessment.

Assessment

- Examination features will depend on the severity of the exacerbation.
- There will be a reduction in the peak expiratory flow rate (PEFR). Most patients will know what their best PEFR is.
- The patient may have tachypnoea, tachycardia (possibly due to overuse of a salbutamol inhaler) and bilateral wheezes on auscultation.
- There may also be features indicative of an underlying trigger such as pyrexia, purulent sputum, coarse crepitations over the affected lung fields; all of which suggest a lower respiratory tract infection.

Management [1], [2]

- The aim is to treat the underlying causes (e.g. antibiotics for bacterial infections), relieve the bronchoconstriction with a bronchodilator (e.g. salbutamol inhaler), and reduce broncho-pulmonary inflammation (e.g. prednisolone 40–50mg PO once daily × 5 days).
- There is no difference in outcomes when comparing salbutamol delivered by a metered dose inhaler and a nebuliser; 4 puffs of a metered dose inhaler actuated in rapid succession at 10-minute intervals is considered to be equivalent to 1.5mg salbutamol nebuliser[3].
- Consider prescribing a proton pump inhibitor (PPI) to reduce the risk of prednisolone-induced gastric erosions.
- Patients should be advised to follow up with their own GP or their asthma nurse to discuss their asthma and consider having a rescue pack at home (oral antibiotics and oral steroids to treat acute infective exacerbations).

Red flag features indicative of status asthmaticus

This is a life-threatening medical emergency, characterised by:

- an inability to complete sentences
- cyanosis
- inability to lie flat
- respiratory rate >25 breaths per minute (normal 12–20)
- recessions
- nasal flaring
- confusion
- silent chest on auscultation
- PEFR <33%
- SpO_2 <92% on air.

Patients should be started on an oxygen-driven nebuliser and given oral or IM steroids.

Status asthmaticus requires an emergency admission via a category 1 or 2 ambulance.

Acute bronchitis

Presentation

- Acute bronchitis presents with a productive cough, chest tightness and wheeze of less than 3 weeks' duration.
- There may be underlying predisposing factors such as a history of smoking tobacco, dust exposure or immunodeficiency.

All but the most well patient will require a face-to-face assessment.

Assessment

- Respiratory examination will reveal bilateral wheezes.
- Severity can be determined by assessing basic observations.
- Low oxygen saturations, tachycardia, tachypnoea, recessions and hypotension are indications for referral to the on-call medical team.

Management [4]

- Most cases are viral in aetiology and tend to resolve with supportive therapy such as fluids, an expectorant linctus, steam and menthol vapour inhalation.
- A salbutamol inhaler will help to relieve bronchoconstriction and oral prednisolone will assist in relieving bronchial inflammation.
- If the patient is systemically unwell or symptoms have been ongoing for more than 7 days, it is prudent to consider a course of oral antibiotics such as amoxicillin 500mg TDS × 5–7 days or clarithromycin 500mg BD × 5–7 days.
- If you do not think an immediate prescription is warranted, consider a delayed prescription if there is a risk of complications due to comorbidities such as diabetes mellitus and chronic cardiac conditions.

- Advise the patient that symptoms should start to resolve after 72 hours. If not, or if symptoms worsen, the patient should seek further medical attention.

Chronic obstructive pulmonary disease (COPD)

Presentation

- This condition encompasses chronic bronchitis and emphysema.
- Patients with COPD will have symptoms that fall within these two entities.
- The diagnosis of COPD will usually have been established earlier in the patient's life.
- There may be a history of smoking tobacco, exposure to inhaled occupational hazards, alpha-1 anti-trypsin deficiency, or congenital lung conditions such as cystic fibrosis, which are all predisposers to developing COPD.
- Infections, both viral and bacterial, tend to be common triggers.

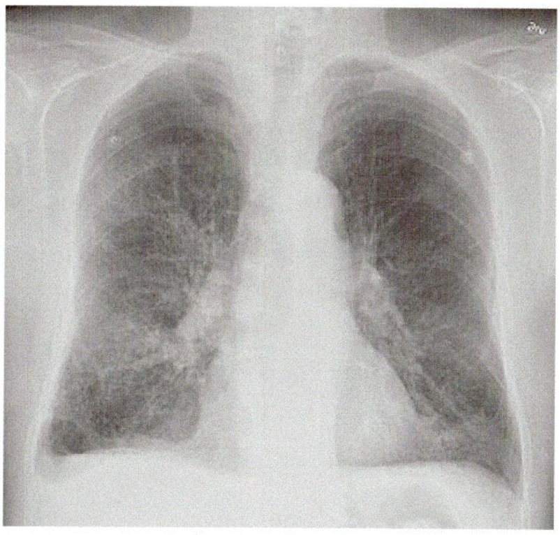

Fig. 8.1: Chest X-ray changes in COPD: hyperinflation, flattening of diaphragm, increased vascular markings.

Reproduced from Häggström, M. (2014) *Wikiversity Journal of Medicine* 1(2). doi:10.15347/wjm/2014.008. CC0 1.0 Universal Public Domain Dedication.

The severity of the exacerbation can often be determined over the phone or via video consultation.

If the patient is unable to complete sentences, is cyanotic, tachypnoeic and has recessions, an emergency ambulance should be arranged.

Some patients may be calling to request an emergency supply of medication to manage the exacerbation, and in such cases a prescription can be sent electronically to the patient's nominated pharmacy. However, if there is any doubt then consider a face-to-face assessment.

Assessment

- The patient will be acutely breathless and may or may not have a productive cough.
- Oxygen saturations may not always be a reliable indicator of the severity of the exacerbation and it is important to assess the respiratory rate and work of breathing.
- The patient may be working extremely hard to maintain their oxygen saturations and will be at risk of fatigue and further respiratory compromise.
- A chest X-ray may exhibit chronic changes associated with COPD (see *Fig. 8.1*), as well as any potential causes of an exacerbation such as pneumonia.

Management

- Management of acute exacerbations is aimed at treating the underlying trigger (antibiotics for bacterial infections), relieving bronchoconstriction (salbutamol inhalers or salbutamol nebuliser 5mg stat and ipratropium nebuliser 0.5mg stat), reducing intrapulmonary and intrabronchial inflammation (prednisolone 30mg × 7–14 days).
- Consider prescribing a PPI (e.g. lansoprazole 15mg OD) with oral corticosteroids to reduce the risk of gastric erosion and gastric bleeding.
- Patients with end-stage COPD have a strong element of anxiety contributing to acute exacerbations. This can be managed with oral anxiolytics such as lorazepam 0.5mg when required; however, these should be prescribed with care as they can suppress breathing.
- Care should be taken when administering supportive oxygen therapy as high doses can suppress breathing further; hence starting off at 2L of oxygen per minute and titrating the dose upwards is appropriate.

Hospital referral criteria for those with acute exacerbations of COPD

Admission to hospital should be considered if the patient is unable to cope at home, has severe dyspnoea, has cyanosis, has peripheral oedema, is confused, has a low GCS, is already on long-term oxygen therapy at home, has a respiratory rate >25 breaths per minute, SpO_2<90% on air or has additional comorbidities, e.g. cardiac impairment.

Pneumonia

Presentation

- Patients may be generally unwell, commonly presenting with shortness of breath, cough and pyrexia.
- Atypical pneumonias will also give rise to extrapulmonary manifestations, an example being mycoplasma pneumonia which can cause a generalised rash.

Although a detailed history can be taken over the phone and the diagnosis can be suspected, a face-to-face assessment may be required to elicit signs of pulmonary consolidation and also to determine the severity of the infection and respiratory compromise.

Assessment [5]

- Findings may include low SpO_2, cyanosis, tachypnoea and tachycardia.
- Bear in mind that young people can look relatively well but will be working hard to maintain oxygen saturations and as a result can 'crash' suddenly.
- Examination of the chest will reveal the following signs on the affected side: decreased expansion, coarse crepitations, decreased breath sounds, bronchial breathing, increased vocal resonance and dullness on percussion.
- The most common cause of community-acquired pneumonia is viral; however, it can be difficult to distinguish a viral pneumonia from a bacterial pneumonia clinically.

- A chest X-ray will show consolidation (*Fig 8.2*). Bear in mind that X-ray changes can lag behind clinical features by a few days and can remain present several weeks after clinical improvement.

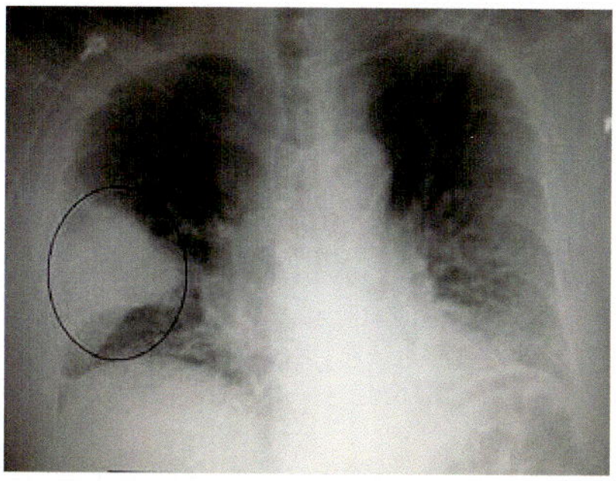

Fig. 8.2: A very prominent pneumonia of the middle lobe of the right lung.

Reproduced from https://commons.wikimedia.org/wiki/File:PneumonisWedge09.JPG under a CC BY-SA 3.0 Unported licence (image by James Heilman, MD).

The severity of community-acquired pneumonia can be assessed using the **CURB-65 score**.

The following factors indicate a poor prognosis: **C**onfusion, a **U**rea >7mmol/L, **R**espiratory rate >30bpm, **B**P systolic <90mmHg or diastolic <60mmHg, age >**65** years.

If two or more of the above factors are present, then the patient should be referred to the on-call medical team. However, in some cases it may be inappropriate, e.g. a 95-year-old in a nursing home with Alzheimer's. In such cases it would be best practice to do what is in the patient's best interests after discussion with their next of kin.

In the community obtaining a serum urea value quickly can be difficult, so the **CRB-65** score can be used and is based solely on clinical assessment.

Prognosis based on the CURB-65 and CRB-65 scores is estimated as follows:

Score 0	= low risk (<1% mortality)
Score 1 or 2	= intermediate risk (1–10% mortality)
Score 3 or 4	= high risk (>10 % mortality).

Management [6], [7]

- Acutely unwell patients should be transferred via ambulance.
- Mild cases of bacterial pneumonia can be managed in the community with oral antibiotics such as amoxicillin 500mg TDS × 5–7 days or doxycycline 100mg 2 capsules on the first day and then 1 capsule a day thereafter for 5–7 days, or clarithromycin 500mg BD × 5–7 days.
- In young patients and smokers consider amoxicillin with clarithromycin, as there is a higher risk of atypical organisms being responsible.
- Recovery from pneumonia can take several weeks; the associated fatigue and malaise can take several months to resolve.
- CXR changes can take up to 28 days to resolve[8].

CURB-65 score can be used to assess prognosis:
C – Confusion
U – Urea >7mmol/L (omit in CRB-65 score)
R – Respiratory rate >30 breaths/min
B – Blood pressure (SBP <90mmHg / DBP <60mmHg)
65 – Age >65 years

Pleurisy

Presentation

- Pleurisy is a common cause of chest pain.
- Onset can be sudden or gradual in nature and it is usually viral in aetiology.
- The pain is nearly always pleuritic in nature and there may be an associated cough.
- Serious underlying causes include:
  - pneumonia, especially pneumococcal pneumonia
  - pulmonary infarction
  - Coxsackie B virus (Bornholm disease)
  - malignancy, e.g. bronchogenic carcinoma
  - lung abscess
  - bronchiectasis
  - asbestos pleural disease, including mesothelioma
  - trauma
  - tuberculosis
  - systemic lupus erythematosus
  - rheumatoid lung disease.

A video consultation may assist in determining if the patient is acutely unwell, in severe pain or has acute dyspnoea. In such cases a category 1 or 2 ambulance should be dispatched.

As most patients with pleurisy will be well, a face-to-face assessment can be arranged for further assessment.

Assessment

- General observations will be within normal limits unless there is underlying pathology.
- Respiratory examination will usually be normal, unless there is serious underlying pathology. Occasionally a pleural rub may be heard over the affected area.

Management

- Provided the patient is well and there are no serious underlying causes, management centres on reassurance, oral anti-inflammatories such as ibuprofen 400mg TDS and deep breathing exercises, e.g. 5 deep breaths 5 times a day for 5 days.
- Symptoms usually settle within 14 days.
- Acutely unwell patients should be referred to the on-call medical team.
- Patients suspected of having serious underlying causes should be referred to their own GP for follow-up assessment and investigations.

Pneumothorax

Presentation

- A pneumothorax is an uncommon presentation in primary care; however, it does require a high index of suspicion which is the key to an early diagnosis.

- Patients may often be young with no underlying lung conditions.
- Predisposing factors include chest trauma, chronic lung disease and connective tissue disorders.
- Presenting features are sharp pleuritic chest pain (often this may radiate to the back or shoulder), dyspnoea and a dry cough.

A pneumothorax cannot be diagnosed over the phone and provided the patient sounds relatively well, a face-to-face assessment can be arranged to elicit clinical signs which suggest a pneumothorax.

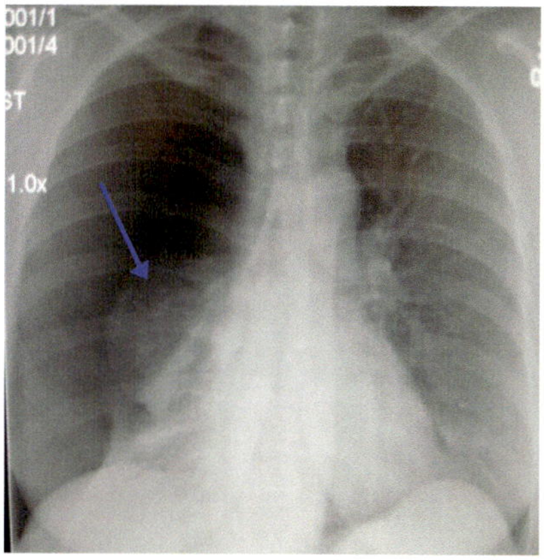

Fig. 8.3: Chest X-ray showing a right-sided pneumothorax.

Reproduced from https://en.wikipedia.org/wiki/Pneumothorax under a CC BY 3.0 licence (image by James Heilman, MD).

Assessment

- The patient may be tachypnoeic with low oxygen saturations; tachycardia may also be present. However, in cases of gradual onset all observations may be within normal range.
- Chest signs include decreased expansion, decreased breath sounds, decreased vocal resonance and hyper-resonance on percussion.
- A chest X-ray (*Fig. 8.3*) will confirm the diagnosis.

Management [9], [10]

- Patients with a pneumothorax where the lung field border is >2cm away from the ribcage should be referred to ED.
- Patients in respiratory distress or those with a tension pneumothorax should also be referred to ED.
- If the patient is well and the pneumothorax is small (<2cm away from the ribcage) then the patient can be monitored in an outpatient setting and followed up with a repeat chest X-ray in 4–6 weeks to ensure resolution.

Pulmonary embolism [11],[12]

Presentation

- This is an important and potentially fatal cause of acute chest pain and dyspnoea.
- There may or may not be obvious risk factors such as a previous history of a PE or a DVT, neoplastic disease, prolonged immobilisation or a clotting diathesis.
- Chest pain tends to be of sudden onset and pleuritic in nature, i.e. worse on deep breathing or coughing.
- There may be associated dyspnoea and/or haemoptysis.
- Patients with a suspected PE should be referred directly to ED.

- If the chest pain or dyspnoea is severe, then transfer should be via a category 1 or 2 ambulance.

A video consultation may assist in assessing the severity of symptoms, especially the dyspnoea.

If the patient is not acutely unwell and it is unclear what the cause of the chest pain is, a face-to-face examination is warranted.

Assessment

- The patient will often have tachypnoea, tachycardia, low SpO_2 (oxygen saturations) and hypotension.
- Auscultation over the affected lung fields may reveal decreased breath sounds and dullness on percussion.
- Bear in mind that clinical examination can sometimes be normal in patients who have a PE.
- A PE can be asymptomatic, and can occasionally be an incidental finding on a CT pulmonary angiogram (CTPA).
- Consider asking the patient to undertake physical activity (e.g. walk 50m); if there is a drop in oxygen saturations this would support the diagnosis of a PE. However, bear in mind that other conditions, such as Covid-19 pneumonitis, can also result in a drop in oxygen saturations after physical activity.

Management

- If a PE is suspected, administer high-flow oxygen and pain relief.
- Referral to ED is mandatory as the patient will require further investigations including a CTPA to confirm or rule out the diagnosis.

Patients with a PE can have normal observations.

Covid-19

Presentation

- This is predominantly a respiratory disease caused by the SARS-CoV-2 virus (a coronavirus).
- The first case was recorded in 2019 in China and due to worldwide spread it has resulted in a global pandemic which is still ongoing at the time of writing. The World Health Organization declared it was no longer a global health emergency in May 2023.
- Symptoms are variable and include: runny nose, headache, fatigue (mild or severe), sneezing, sore throat. Approximately one-third of infected people will not have any symptoms[13].
- As newer variants of the SARS-Cov-2 virus have emerged and as the worldwide vaccination programme has progressed, symptom variability has evolved, with some people reporting cold-like symptoms only.
- Gastrointestinal symptoms such as diarrhoea and vomiting tend to be more common in children.

- Lung involvement will result in dyspnoea, hypoxia, haemoptysis, respiratory failure.
- Risk factors for severe disease include: advanced age (over 70 years), frailty, immunocompromise, being unvaccinated for Covid-19, the presence of chronic medical problems such as heart disease, lung disease and diabetes mellitus.
- The overall mortality rate is 1%[14].

In all patients suspected of having a SARS-CoV-2 infection a detailed history should be taken over the phone, with particular attention being paid to the presence of risk factors.

Patients suspected of having a SARS-CoV-2 infection should be encouraged to confirm the diagnosis via PCR (polymerase chain reaction) testing, which is available in the UK by telephoning 119 or via the www.gov.uk website. Alternatively, patients can undertake a rapid antigen test at home; test kits are available from local pharmacies. Patients who test positive and have mild symptoms should be advised to isolate for the recommended number of days and can be managed at home with supportive measures.

Isolation periods will vary by country and region, and as the general population gains immunity through exposure to the virus and through vaccination, it is anticipated that isolation periods will be reduced in duration and may eventually end. The reader is advised to check local and government guidance.

A video consultation may help in trying to ascertain the severity of symptoms.

Patients who are suspected of having pneumonia or pneumonitis (severe dyspnoea, increased respiratory rate, hypoxia) should be assessed face-to-face; this should ideally be done in an isolation room or at a Covid Hub; these are specific areas within hospitals and OOH clinics to assess patients with Covid-19 or those suspected to have Covid-19.

Assessment

- This should be undertaken with appropriate PPE.
- Assess vital signs, especially oxygen saturations; a reading <92% with an increased respiratory rate is associated with increased mortality[15].
- Other features which suggest severe disease include haemoptysis, cyanosis, mottled skin, confusion, being difficult to rouse, collapse[16].
- Assess for potential complications such as a PE or superimposed bacterial pneumonia.

Management

- Patients with mild symptoms should be advised to isolate if necessary and in accordance with local and national guidance.
- Advise the patient of potential complications to look out for and to seek further medical attention if they occur.
- Pyrexia can be managed with paracetamol and ibuprofen.
- Avoiding lying supine and taking pholcodine linctus, available over the counter, can help with the cough.
- Advise the patient to remain well hydrated.
- Patients at high risk of hospitalisation (e.g. immunocompromised) should be considered for antiviral medication medication such as sotrovimab and molnupiravir[17].

  - sotrovimab is a neutralising monoclonal antibody agent which is given as a one-off dose of 500mg IV. It can be given in the community and has been shown to reduce the risk of hospitalisation by 85%[17].
  - an alternative antiviral agent is molnupiravir which can be taken orally; the recommended dose is 800mg every 12 hours × 5 days. Treatment should be started within the first 5 days of symptoms[17].
  - Paxlovid (brand name of nirmatrelvir and ritonavir) is also available on prescription. 300mg (two pink tablets) and 100mg (one white tablet) are taken twice daily for 5 days. Treatment should be started within the first 5 days of symptoms.
- Patients should be referred to the Covid Medicines Delivery Unit in accordance with local guidance and your employing organisation's protocol.
- Treat any superimposed bacterial infections such as pneumonia with appropriate oral antibiotics.
- Patients with severe disease, or at risk of developing severe disease and those unable to care for themselves, should be referred to hospital for consideration of oxygen therapy, antiviral drugs, monoclonal antibodies, dexamethasone, and the management of complications such as acute renal failure.
- For patients who are elderly, frail, with extensive comorbidities and in whom escalation of management would be inappropriate, consider palliative care.
- As Covid-19 is a relatively new illness, prescribing guidance and policies are evolving and therefore it would be appropriate to discuss treatment options with a specialist and also to consult the most up-to-date guidance.

Summary for respiratory

- Status asthmaticus is a life-threatening condition.
- Always assess inhaler technique, as poor technique can be a cause of poor asthma control.
- End-stage COPD patients may have a strong element of anxiety contributing to their breathlessness.
- The CURB-65 and CRB-65 scores can be used to assess prognosis in patients with pneumonia.
- PE must be ruled out when assessing patients presenting with acute chest pain.
- Patients who have a PE can have normal observations, so if there is a high index of suspicion refer to ED.

References

1. British Thoracic Society (2019) *British guideline on the management of asthma*. A national clinical guideline. Available at: www.brit-thoracic.org.uk/quality-improvement/guidelines/asthma/

2. NICE (no date) *Asthma, acute*. Available at: https://bnf.nice.org.uk/treatment-summary/asthma-acute.html

3. Rodrigo, G. and Rodrigo, C. (1993) Comparison of salbutamol delivered by nebulizer or metered-dose inhaler with a pear-shaped space in acute asthma. *Current Therapeutic Research*, **54(6):** 797–808.

4. NICE (2019) *Cough (acute): antimicrobial prescribing* [NG120]. Available at: www.nice.org.uk/guidance/ng120

5. NICE (updated 2023) *Pneumonia in adults: diagnosis and management* [CG191]. Available at: www.nice.org.uk/guidance/cg191

6. British Thoracic Society (2015) *Annotated BTS Guideline for the management of CAP in adults*. Summary of recommendations. Available at: www.brit-thoracic.org.uk/quality-improvement/guidelines/pneumonia-adults/

7. NICE (2019) *Pneumonia (community-acquired): antimicrobial prescribing* [NG138]. Available at: www.nice.org.uk/guidance/ng138

8. Bruns, A.H, Oosterheert, J.J., El Moussaoui, R. *et al.* (2009) Pneumonia recovery; discrepancies in perspectives of the radiologist, physician and patient. *J Gen Intern Med*, **25(3):** 203–206.

9. MacDuff, A., Arnold, A. and Harvey, J. (2010) Management of spontaneous pneumothorax: British Thoracic Society pleural disease guideline 2010. *Thorax*, **65:** ii18–ii31.

10. Kaneda, H., Nakano, T., Taniguchi, Y. *et al.* (2013) Three-step management of pneumothorax: time for a re-think on initial management. *Interact Cardiovasc Thorac Surg*, **16(2):** 186–192.

11. Riedel, M. (2001) Acute pulmonary embolism 1: pathophysiology, clinical presentation, and diagnosis. *Heart*, **85:** 229–240.

12. Miniati, M., Cenci, C., Monti, S. and Poli, D. (2012) Clinical presentation of acute pulmonary embolism: survey of 800 cases. *PLoS One*, **7(2):** e30891.

13. Oran, D.P. and Topol, E.J. (2021) The proportion of SARS-CoV-2 infections that are asymptomatic: a systematic review. *Annals of Internal Medicine*, **174(5):** 655–662.

14. NICE (revised 2024) *Coronavirus – COVID-19*. Available at: https://cks.nice.org.uk/topics/coronavirus-covid-19

15. Chatterjee, N.A., Jensen, P.N., Harris, A.W. *et al.* (2021) Admission respiratory status predicts mortality in COVID-19. *Influenza and Other Respiratory Viruses*. Available at: https://onlinelibrary.wiley.com/doi/10.1111/irv.12869

16. NICE (updated 2024) *COVID-19 rapid guideline: managing COVID-19* [NG191]. Available at: www.nice.org.uk/guidance/ng191/chapter/Recommendations

17. Department of Health & Social Care (2021) *Interim Clinical Commissioning Policy: Neutralising monoclonal antibodies and intravenous antivirals in the treatment of COVID-19 in hospitalised patients*. Available at: www.cas.mhra.gov.uk/ViewandAcknowledgment/ViewAttachment.aspx?Attachment_id=103882

9

Chapter 9: **Neurology**

"With the nervous system intact the reactions of the various parts of that system, the 'simple reflexes', are ever combined into great unitary harmonies, actions which in their sequence one upon another constitute in their continuity what may be termed the 'behaviour'."
Charles Scott Sherrington

Assessment of patients presenting with acute neurological conditions

Telephone

- A detailed history can be taken over the phone.
- Red flag features (see below) can be identified over the phone and patients can be referred directly to ED.
- The two most common types of headaches are migraines and tension-type headaches, and these can often be diagnosed on the history alone.
- Sudden onset of a severe occipital headache with neurological features is suggestive of a subarachnoid haemorrhage.
- If there is any doubt as to the aetiology of the headaches, a face-to-face assessment should be arranged.
- Ipsilateral limb and facial weakness is due to a stroke until proven otherwise, and patients who present with this on the phone should have an emergency ambulance transfer to hospital.

Face-to-face

- Always assess and record general observations.
- When assessing patients with headaches it is essential to record negative findings, especially neck stiffness and photophobia, as well as the presence or absence of a rash or a high temperature.
- Presenting your negative findings to your patient may also help with reassurance.
- A full neurological examination may be required, which may assist in reassuring anxious patients.

Key red flag features of headaches

- Sudden onset
- Neurological deficit (e.g. limb weakness)
- Associated rashes
- Neck stiffness
- Photophobia
- A history of significant trauma.

Patients with these features should be referred to ED or the on-call medical team.

Tension-type headaches

Presentation

- The pain is often described as a tight band across the head, or a pressure on top of the head.
- The pain may originate from or radiate to the neck and shoulder girdle.
- These types of headaches tend to be chronic and the patient will usually have had them in the past.

Video consultation may be helpful, and in certain circumstances a crude neurological examination, assessing for neck stiffness and limb weakness, can be undertaken.

A face-to-face assessment will be required if there are any doubts as to the cause of the headache, to assess for focal neurological deficits and possibly to reassure the patient.

Assessment

- It is worth asking about possible psychological and emotional stress factors, as most patients will be able to make the link between these and the headaches.
- Observations will be within normal range.
- Conducting a full neurological examination can assist with reassurance.

Management

- Tension-type headaches are managed with rest, addressing the underlying stress factors and relaxation techniques.
- Short-term relief from the pain can be achieved with simple analgesia, including paracetamol and ibuprofen.
- Patients should be advised to follow up with their own GP, should the headaches persist.

Migraines

Presentation

- Most patients who present in an urgent care or OOH GP setting will have an established diagnosis of migraines.

- The pain is usually described as a pounding sensation arising from within the head; this is in contrast to tension-type headaches, where the pain is usually described as a pressure on top of the head or a band around the head.
- Common triggers include stress, bright lights, hypoglycaemia, alcohol and foods such as chocolate and cheese.
- The patient may or may not experience visual aura prior to the onset.
- Associated features include nausea, vomiting, photophobia, hyperacusis, speech disturbances and hemiparesis.

Video consultation will usually be of limited value.

A face-to-face assessment will be required if there are any doubts as to the cause of the headache, to assess for focal neurological deficits and possibly to reassure the patient.

Assessment

- Clinical examination will be normal unless there are associated complications such as hemiparesis.
- It is important to record examination findings along with the absence or presence of red flag features (see red flag box).

Management [1],[2]

- Management is centred on reassurance, keeping well hydrated, regular meals, a healthy diet, analgesia and avoiding triggers.
- Oral analgesia options are:
  - paracetamol 1g every 6 hours with ibuprofen 400mg every 8 hours
  - aspirin 900mg as a one-off dose
  - sumatriptan 50–100mg when needed
  - amitriptyline 10mg at night
  - propranolol 40mg every 8 hours or 160mg modified release once a day.
- Anti-emetics such as cyclizine 50mg every 8 hours will also help with nausea and vomiting.
- If nausea and vomiting is severe, medication may have to be administered rectally, IM or SC.
- Avoid codeine and other opiates as these are associated with rebound headaches.
- Patients suffering from frequent debilitating migraines should be referred to their GP to discuss prophylactic medication.

Meningitis

Meningitis is a separate entity to meningococcal septicaemia; it refers to inflammation of the meninges and on its own will not present with a rash.

Presentation

- There is usually an insidious onset of a high temperature, headache, nausea and vomiting.

A face-to-face assessment should be undertaken in all patients who have a headache and a high temperature and no other obvious cause for symptoms.

Assessment

- Characteristically there will be neck stiffness, photophobia and a positive Kernig's sign (hip flexed, knee extended from 90° causes pain) confirming irritation of the meninges.
- A full examination including assessment of vital signs should be undertaken.
- A neurological examination looking for any focal neurological deficits should be conducted.
- There are various causes including viruses, bacteria, fungi and drugs.

Management

- Most cases are viral and tend to be self-limiting.
- It can be difficult to distinguish causes clinically and patients with suspected meningitis should be referred to hospital, as some causes can result in serious sequelae and death.

Subarachnoid haemorrhage (SAH)

Presentation[3]

- The patient will be relatively young (<60 years of age).
- The key characteristic features are the sudden onset and severity of the headache along with the location, which is the back of the head.
- Frequently patients describe a feeling of 'being hit on the back of a head with a baseball bat'.
- 50% of patients will have associated loss of consciousness or a seizure.

The sudden onset, location and the severity of the headache is usually enough to suspect the possibility of a SAH. For these reasons patients can be referred directly to ED via an ambulance.

If there is doubt, the history is unclear and the patient is relatively well, a face-to-face assessment can be considered to assess the patient further.

Assessment

- Commonly there is neck stiffness and photophobia.
- A positive Kernig's sign will usually be present 3 hours after the onset of the headache.
- Some patients will have an associated neurological deficit such as a hemiparesis with abnormal plantar responses (extensor).
- Vitreous haemorrhages may also occur.

Management

- All patients with a suspected SAH should be referred immediately to the on-call medical team or ED for an urgent CT scan and lumbar puncture.

Kernig's sign: the patient lies flat on their back, the thigh is flexed at a right angle to the trunk and the knee joint extended. If this causes pain in the back or neck, it is positive and is a feature of meningeal irritation.

Bell's palsy

Presentation

- Bell's palsy is characterised by the sudden onset of unilateral facial weakness (*Fig. 9.1*).
- It is believed it is due to a localised infection from the herpes virus which causes a lower motor neurone weakness of the 7th cranial nerve.

Although the diagnosis can be suspected over the phone, a face-to-face assessment is recommended to ensure there is no frontal sparing and there is no limb involvement. A video consultation may allow this; however, a detailed examination of the skin for herpes zoster lesions will not be possible on video consultation.

A face-to-face assessment can also assist in identifying any potential causes as well as reassuring the patient, as Bell's palsy can often be an alarming condition.

Assessment

- It is important to look in the ears, as the presence of vesicles on the ipsilateral side of the palsy is indicative of Ramsay Hunt syndrome.
- It is important to examine for a parotid gland mass, as this could represent a neoplastic lesion of the parotid gland causing compression of the cranial nerve.
- Characteristically there is no frontal sparing and importantly no limb weakness; hence distinguishing Bell's palsy from a cerebrovascular accident.
- The diagnosis of Bell's palsy is usually a clinical one, unless there is suspicion of another cause.
- 1% of patients who have Bell's palsy will have bilateral facial paralysis.

Management[4]

- Treatment is with high-dose oral prednisolone 50mg OD × 10 days or 60mg × 5 days and then reducing by 10mg a day for another 5 days (total treatment for 10 days).
- Although there is mixed evidence on the efficacy of oral aciclovir, this can be prescribed. A common regime is 800mg PO 5 times a day × 7 days.
- Also consider prescribing a PPI to reduce the risk of prednisolone-induced gastric erosions.
- Patients who are unable to protect the eye should be referred to the ophthalmology clinic and advised to start lubricating eye drops, which are available from the pharmacy.
- A general rule of thumb is that one-third will undergo a complete recovery, one-third will undergo a partial recovery and one-third will be left with unilateral facial paralysis.

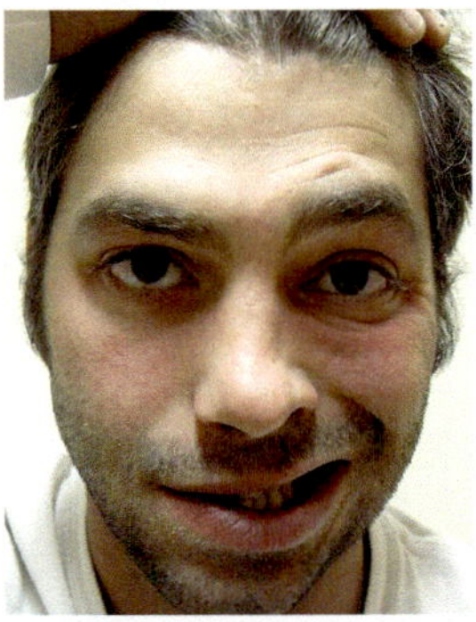

Fig. 9.1: Bell's palsy.

Reproduced from https://commons.wikimedia.org/wiki/File:Bellspalsy.JPG under a CC BY-SA 3.0 licence (photo by James Heilman, MD).

With Bell's palsy there is no frontal sparing, i.e. all the muscles of the affected side of the face are paralysed. This is in contrast to facial weakness caused by a stroke, where the forehead and brow muscles will still be able to move.

Transient global amnesia (TGA)

Presentation

- TGA results in temporary loss of short-term memory; an episode can last up to 8 hours.
- It is usually reported by a witness, with the patient unable to recall any recent events.
- Precipitators include vigorous exercise, temperature changes and stress.
- Patients may have a history of emotional instability, anxiety or depression.

A face-to-face assessment will be required to undertake a neurological examination and to check observations including blood glucose levels.

Assessment

- There is no cognitive disruption and patients will be alert and appear well.
- Recollection of recent events will be affected.
- Affected patients may struggle to form new memories for a short period of time.

Management

- Complete resolution is expected within 24 hours.
- There is no treatment.
- Underlying factors, such as anxiety and stress, should be addressed.

Cerebrovascular accident (CVA)

Presentation

- A CVA presents with sudden and painless onset of facial and limb weakness, altered sensation, speech and swallowing difficulties.
- There will often, but not always, be underlying risk factors such as hypertension, diabetes mellitus, coronary artery disease or peripheral vascular disease.
- Patients may lose consciousness (something not associated with transient ischaemic events).

A face-to-face assessment is rarely required, as the diagnosis will be apparent over the phone. Often the 111 call handler will have raised an ambulance, and telephone triage will not be required.

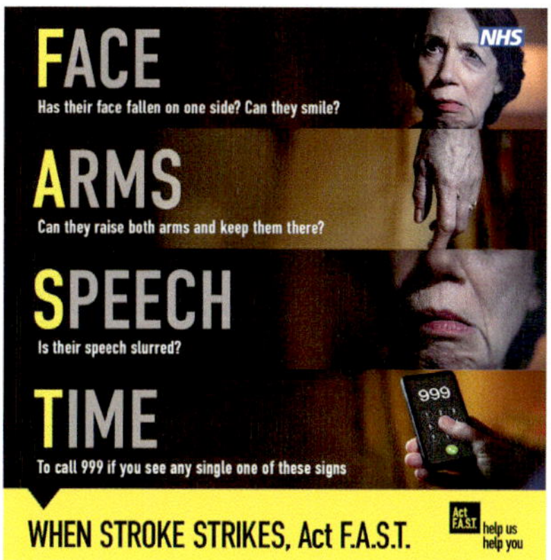
NHS
FACE
Has their face fallen on one side? Can they smile?
ARMS
Can they raise both arms and keep them there?
SPEECH
Is their speech slurred?
TIME
999
To call 999 if you see any single one of these signs
WHEN STROKE STRIKES, Act F.A.S.T.
help us help you

Fig. 9.2: When stroke strikes, act FAST.

Reproduced under an Open Government licence.

Management

- As soon as a stroke is suspected (*Fig. 9.2*), a category 1 or 2 ambulance should be arranged and the patient transferred to the nearest stroke centre or ED.
- If you are with the patient, consider giving aspirin 300mg as a stat dose with gastroprotection (provided there are no contraindications) whilst the ambulance is on its way.
- Patients who are suspected of having had a TIA (transient ischaemic attack) should be started on aspirin 300mg with gastroprotection and referred to a TIA clinic for an assessment within 24 hours.

Trigeminal neuralgia

Presentation

- This can affect any of the three sensory branches of the trigeminal nerve (ophthalmic, maxillary and mandibular).
- The pain is characteristically lancing or piercing in nature, coming in waves.
- The skin over the affected area may feel extremely sensitive or numb.

To a certain extent trigeminal neuralgia is a diagnosis of exclusion and in the majority of cases it will be made on the history and once other causes of facial pain have been excluded. For this reason the diagnosis will be apparent over the phone. A video or face-to-face consultation will assist in excluding other causes such as otitis media or herpes zoster.

Assessment

- There may be altered sensation.
- There will be no motor weakness, and general observations will be within normal range.
- The appearance of vesicles on the skin raises the suspicion of shingles, so a close examination of the scalp and face is essential.

Management

- This is focused on controlling the pain.
- Opiates have been shown to reduce neuropathic pain by one-third, so agents such as codeine can be used in conjunction with more conventional neuropathic pain relief such as amitriptyline 10mg nocte, carbamazepine 200mg BD or gabapentin 100mg TDS (titrated up slowly)[5].
- Patients should be advised to follow up with their own GP.

Cauda equina syndrome

Presentation

- There may be a history of trauma, tumours, inflammatory conditions, infections or spinal stenosis, all of which are predisposing factors.

- Always think of cord compression in patients presenting with back pain or limb symptoms who have an active or past medical history of neoplastic disease.
- It is important to remember not all patients will have back pain; cauda equina syndrome can be painless.

Assessment

- Common features include pain (radiating down the legs), bowel and/or bladder disturbances, altered gait, limb weakness, saddle anaesthesia, loss of sensation in the lower limbs and absent lower limb reflexes.
- Clinical diagnosis can be difficult, as symptoms and signs can evolve and progress over days depending on the underlying aetiology; hence the full gamut of features may not be present at the time of initial assessment.
- Cauda equina syndrome and cord compression are medical emergencies and patients must be referred to on-call spinal surgeons or ED for immediate MRI scans and decompression surgery if indicated.
- Delayed referral can result in permanent neurological deficit and disability.
- One of the most common causes of litigation is due to a failed or delayed diagnosis of cauda equina syndrome[6].

Features of cauda equina syndrome

- Possible risk factors – e.g. trauma, cancer
- Back pain (not always present)
- Bowel disturbances
- Bladder disturbances
- Paraesthesia or anaesthesia affecting the lower limbs
- Saddle anaesthesia
- Loss of anal sphincter tone
- Lower limb motor weakness
- Loss of sensation in the lower limbs
- Absent motor reflexes in the lower limbs

All the features may not be present at the time of assessment.

Summary for neurology

- The most common types of chronic headaches are tension-type headaches and migraines, which share a common management plan.
- Avoid opiates in people with chronic headaches as these can cause rebound headaches.
- Be aware of red flag features associated with headaches; these include sudden onset, neurological deficit (e.g. limb weakness), associated rashes, neck stiffness, photophobia and a history of significant trauma.
- Sudden onset of an occipital headache – think subarachnoid haemorrhage.
- Meningitis does not present with a rash; meningococcal septicaemia presents with a rash.

- Facial and limb weakness is due to a stroke until proven otherwise.
- Pain is not always present with cauda equina syndrome.
- Features of cauda equina syndrome can develop over time and the whole gamut of features may not be apparent at the time of presentation.

References

1. NICE (revised 2024) *Migraine*. Available at: https://cks.nice.org.uk/migraine

2. BNF (no date) *Acute Migraine Treatment*. Available at: https://bnf.nice.org.uk/treatment-summary/migraine.html

3. de Rooij, N.K., Linn, F.H., van der Plas, J.A. *et al.* (2007) Incidence of subarachnoid haemorrhage: a systematic review with emphasis on region, age, gender and time trends. *J Neurol Neurosurg Psychiatry*, **78(12):** 1365–72.

4. NICE (revised 2023) *Bell's palsy management*. Available at: https://cks.nice.org.uk/bells-palsy

5. NICE (revised 2024) *Management of trigeminal neuralgia*. Available at: https://cks.nice.org.uk/trigeminal-neuralgia#!scenario

6. MDU (2017) *Why are unscheduled or out of hours consultations more risky?*

10

Chapter 10: **Endocrinology**

"The doctor of the future will no longer treat the human frame with drugs, but rather will cure and prevent disease with nutrition."
Thomas A. Edison

Assessment of patients presenting with acute metabolic and endocrine conditions

Telephone

- Take a detailed history.
- Enquire about previous episodes and how they were managed.
- Enquire about pre-existing medical conditions.
- Enquire about compliance with medication and results of any recent blood investigations.
- Enquire about any observations and recent capillary blood glucose levels.
- Assess for possible precipitating factors such as infections.

In patients who are acutely unwell with a metabolic condition a face-to-face assessment is rarely required; in the majority of cases an ambulance should be arranged.

Face-to-face

Face-to-face assessments should be considered:

- If the patient has mild symptoms and the diagnosis is unclear.
- If further assessment such as urinalysis is required.
- To assess and treat a precipitating condition.

Hypoglycaemia

Presentation

- This occurs when blood glucose levels fall below 4mmol/L.
- The patient may be on insulin or taking oral hypoglycaemic agents.
- Prolonged fasting and eating disorders are also predisposing conditions.
- Patients with hypoglycaemia will be acutely unwell, semi-conscious, sweating and lethargic.

Often the diagnosis will be apparent on the phone; pre-existing diabetic patients may have a glucometer and will be able to check their own blood glucose.

Patients or carers of those affected should be advised to give the patient a high oral glucose load immediately.

Assessment

- The patient will look unwell with pallor, diaphoresis and lethargy.
- There will be tachycardia and hypovolaemia; a capillary blood glucose will confirm the diagnosis.
- It is good practice to check the blood glucose levels in all patients who are acutely unwell or in severe pain.

Management[1]

- A high glucose load should be administered immediately in the form of a glucose gel or tablets.
- If this is unavailable then any high glucose load such as honey, carbonated soft drinks or a glass of milk or water with 10–15g of sugar can be given orally.
- Patients should be referred to ED for assessment and monitoring.
- Patients with diabetes mellitus should always have their blood glucose levels checked as part of their overall assessment.

Diabetic ketoacidosis (DKA) and hyperosmolar hyperglycaemic non-ketotic (HONK) state

Presentation and assessment[2]

- These are life-threatening emergencies.
- DKA occurs due to a lack of insulin; as a result glucose cannot be utilised as an energy source and instead the liver breaks down fat into ketones to use as energy. The excessive ketones result in the blood and urine becoming acidic.
- In HONK (sometimes referred to as hyperosmolar hyperglycaemic state (HHS)) there is still enough insulin to prevent ketogenesis; however, persistently elevated levels of glucose in the blood and urine result in osmotic diuresis and electrolyte disturbances.
- Both DKA and HONK coexist and the presenting features of both are similar.
- Patients may or may not have been diagnosed with diabetes mellitus in the past and occasionally patients with undiagnosed diabetes mellitus will present with DKA.
- Severe abdominal pain can often be a presenting feature of DKA, and it is important to check blood glucose levels in all patients who are in severe pain.
- Typical presenting features include confusion, lethargy, vomiting, visual disturbances, dehydration, ketotic breath in DKA (often described as smelling of pear drops), hyperventilation or deep laboured breathing, tachycardia, hypotension and coma (due to cerebral oedema).
- Precipitating factors include poor compliance with medication, infection, stress, medication, and acute medical conditions such as pancreatitis.
- A 'HI' reading on the glucometer and the presence of ketones (may not be present in HONK) in the urine will confirm the diagnosis.
- Bear in mind that type I diabetics with DKA may have a normal capillary blood glucose reading.

Management

- IV fluids should be administered if possible and a category 1 or 2 ambulance transfer arranged to ED.

Features of DKA and HONK

- Confusion
- Lethargy
- Vomiting
- Visual disturbances
- Dehydration
- Ketotic breath (in DKA)
- Hyperventilation or deep laboured breathing
- Tachycardia
- Hypotension
- Coma

Addison's disease (adrenal insufficiency) and Addisonian crisis

Presentation

- This is characterised by a lack of adrenal hormones, most notably aldosterone and cortisol.
- Presenting complaints include fatigue, muscle weakness, myalgia, anorexia, low mood, polydipsia, hyperpigmentation, abdominal pain, salt cravings and hypoglycaemia.
- As symptoms are non-specific, a high index of suspicion is required.
- The diagnosis is made on blood investigations including blood electrolyte, blood glucose and serum cortisol levels.
- Patients who present in an OOH setting may well have an established diagnosis and are calling to request advice on how to manage their medication (hydrocortisone and fludrocortisone) during a concurrent illness.
- Addisonian crisis is a life-threatening complication presenting with severe dehydration, sweating, tachypnoea, headache, abdominal pain and severe drowsiness.

Patients who are relatively well and require telephone advice can be provided with this over the phone. If Addisonian crisis is suspected, an emergency admission to hospital via ambulance should be arranged.

Assessment

- Always check general observations including a blood glucose level.
- Patients with Addisonian crisis will be pale, cold, clammy, tachypnoeic, tachycardic and hypotensive.

Management[3]

- Advise patients with mild to moderate intercurrent illness to double the dose of their hydrocortisone until recovery, ensure adequate hydration and avoid becoming hypoglycaemic by having small frequent meals.

- Advise patients with severe illness to take 100mg of hydrocortisone via their emergency injection and refer to hospital.
- For patients with suspected Addisonian crisis, administer 100mg of hydrocortisone IM or IV and commence intravenous rehydration. Refer the patient immediately to hospital via a category 1 or 2 ambulance.

Summary for endocrinology

- All patients including children who are acutely and systemically unwell should have their blood glucose levels checked.
- Patients with suspected Addisonian crisis should be referred to hospital via emergency ambulance.

References

1. BNF (no date) *Hypoglycaemia – treatment of hypoglycaemia*. Available at: https://bnf.nice.org.uk/treatment-summary/hypoglycaemia.html

2. BNF (no date) *Diabetic hyperglycaemic emergencies*. Available at: https://bnf.nice.org.uk/treatment-summary/diabetic-hyperglycaemic-emergencies.html

3. NICE (revised 2024) *Addison's disease – management*. Available at: https://cks.nice.org.uk/topics/addisons-disease/management/

11

Chapter 11: **Gastroenterology**

"An army marches on its stomach."
Napoleon Bonaparte

Assessment of patients presenting with acute gastrointestinal conditions

Telephone

- A detailed history can be taken over the phone.
- The patient's age can be an important factor when determining the aetiology; for example, diverticulitis is more common in the elderly and appendicitis is more common in the younger patient.
- Enquire about systemic symptoms and the possibility of red flag features such as coffee ground vomitus, which suggests upper gastrointestinal (GI) bleeding.
- Beware of pain radiating beyond the abdomen, e.g. GORD causing chest pain.
- Consider non-GI pathology, e.g. aortic dissection as a cause of abdominal pain.
- For patients who have severe abdominal pain and seem to be acutely unwell, consider a direct transfer to hospital via an emergency ambulance.
- A video consultation may help to determine the severity of the pain the patient is in and whether they are generally unwell.

Face-to-face

Face-to-face assessments should be considered in the following circumstances:

- The diagnosis is unclear.
- A physical examination is required to confirm the diagnosis, for example in patients with severe ano-rectal pain.
- Further investigations such as a urinalysis may help in determining the cause.
- In the young and elderly, as there is an increased possibility of serious pathology being the cause of the symptoms and also the risk of complications is higher.
- It is important to examine inguinal orifices to rule out herniae and associated complications such as incarceration (painful, tender, irreducible and loss of cough impulse).
- Also consider a testicular examination in male patients, as testicular pathology can present as abdominal pain.

Gastro-oesophageal reflux disease (GORD)

Presentation

- Usually there is a protracted history, often weeks or months of symptoms.
- Most patients will self-proclaim the diagnosis.
- There may be obvious predisposing factors (often unbeknownst to the patient) such as obesity, constipation, tobacco consumption, excessive alcohol consumption, NSAID use and a liking for spicy foods.
- Also one should not underestimate the effect of stress on precipitating GORD and dyspepsia.
- A detailed enquiry will usually result in the patient admitting to some of the aforementioned predisposing factors.
- Symptoms will frequently be related to food and fluid intake, often being exacerbated by some foods and relieved by others.
- Typical symptoms include a retrosternal or epigastric burning or discomfort with belching, bloating, nausea and water brash (excessive salivation due to GORD).

The diagnosis will often be apparent over the phone or on video consultation. A face-to-face assessment is rarely required but may be warranted if there is high patient anxiety or if there are red flag features (see below).

Assessment

- Clinical examination is normal and the patient is usually comfortable at rest.

Management

- This is centred on controlling predisposing factors, lifestyle changes and medication such as alginates (e.g. Gaviscon), H_2 receptor antagonists (e.g. famotidine), and PPIs (e.g. pantoprazole).
- Many of these are available to purchase at pharmacies.

Key red flag features to enquire about for GORD

Persistent symptoms despite treatment; vomiting; weight loss; new onset in the elderly.

The presence of these warrants further investigations such as a gastroscopy or CT imaging.

Predisposers for GORD

- Certain foods (coffee, alcohol, fatty / spicy foods)
- Being overweight
- Smoking
- Stress
- Medicines (e.g. NSAIDs)

Lifestyle changes to manage GORD

- Address predisposers
- Smaller, more frequent meals
- Exercise
- Try to lose weight
- Sleep with extra pillows
- Avoid eating within 3–4 hours of bedtime

Oesophageal rupture

Presentation

- This is rare, with most cases being iatrogenic in aetiology.
- Occasionally this can be due to excessive vomiting; when this occurs it is termed Boerhaave's syndrome.
- Patients will present with severe chest and upper abdominal pain.
- Dyspnoea will be marked and the patient will struggle to speak in complete sentences.
- The onset of circulatory collapse is rapid.

Patients with suspected oesophageal rupture should have an emergency ambulance called out to them immediately.

Assessment

- There will be associated odynophagia, tachycardia, tachypnoea and pyrexia.
- At the time of presentation the patient may already be in hypovolaemic shock.
- The presence of chest pain, vomiting and subcutaneous emphysema (termed Mackler's triad) is present in only 14% of patients who have oesophageal rupture.

Management

- This is a medical emergency; the mortality rate is exceptionally high.
- A CT scan is usually required to confirm the diagnosis.
- Any patients with suspected oesophageal rupture should be transferred via an emergency ambulance to ED.

Mallory–Weiss tear

Presentation

- This refers to a tear or break in the mucosa of the oesophagus.
- Precipitators are recurrent retching, vomiting, coughing or straining.
- The bleeding will be bright red and small in volume.
- Pain is not always present.

A face-to-face assessment is rarely required as the patient will be well and the diagnosis can be made on the history.

Occasionally a video consultation may assist in alleviating any patient anxiety and assisting the clinician in confirming the patient is well.

Assessment

- The patient will be generally well and observations will be within normal limits.

Management

- The patient should be reassured that the pain and bleeding will settle; anti-emetics will help with nausea and vomiting.
- Antacids may also help alleviate any pain associated with gastro-oesophageal reflux.

Acute appendicitis

Presentation

- Acute appendicitis will usually affect people between the ages of 4 and 40 years of age.
- The lifetime risk is 7–8%[1].
- It is more common in males.
- Pain tends to be of gradual onset, often starting around the umbilicus.
- Over the course of 48 to 72 hours it will tend to become more localised to the right iliac fossa. Occasionally pain can be of relatively sudden onset, with symptoms progressing rapidly over 24 hours.
- Loss of appetite is a characteristic feature and the 'Hamburger' test (especially in children) can be helpful in ascertaining loss of appetite[2]. If a patient refuses their favourite food then this is considered 80% sensitive for anorexia, an associated feature of acute appendicitis.
- Nausea and vomiting are also usually present.

Ideally a face-to-face assessment is required to assess the patient and also rule out the possibility of an alternative diagnosis; however, on some occasions a patient may have appropriate diagnostic equipment at home and therefore may be able to check basic observations.

If there is a competent adult with the patient, they may be able to undertake an abdominal examination and elicit tenderness over McBurney's point, thereby supporting the diagnosis of acute appendicitis. In the past I have diagnosed appendicitis via video consultation, and a direct referral to the general surgeons and subsequent surgery confirmed the presence of an acutely necrotic appendix. However, if there is any doubt a face-to-face assessment should be requested.

Assessment

- Clinical examination involves checking basic observations and also a urine dipstick test to rule out a urinary tract infection (the general surgeons will nearly always ask the results of this if you are considering referring the patient to them).
- Also check blood glucose levels, as diabetic ketoacidosis can present with acute abdominal pain.

- Typically the patient will have tenderness over McBurney's point (located one-third of the distance from the anterior superior iliac spine to the umbilicus) with rebound tenderness and guarding.
- Bowel sounds will be present and a rectal examination will be normal.

Management [1]

- If the patient is relatively well and the diagnosis unclear then one may adopt a wait and watch regime; however, safety-netting is vital. Consider arranging a second contact in 6–8 hours' time to follow up the patient.
- A raised white cell count can support the diagnosis but is non-specific.
- True appendicitis will progress and the pain will become worse.
- Patients with acute appendicitis should be referred to the on-call surgeons.

Diarrhoea and vomiting

Presentation

- The majority of cases will be due to viral gastroenteritis and therefore be self-limiting, lasting no more than 7 days.
- There may be a history of travel or patients may be able to attribute it to certain foods or a night out where a suspect kebab or burger was consumed, sometimes knowingly!
- A detailed history can assist in identifying those at risk of dehydration.
- Ask about the number of episodes of vomiting and diarrhoea over a 24-hour period. Persistent vomiting over 24 hours puts the patient at risk of dehydration.
- Ask about the time of the last episode of vomiting and diarrhoea – if the patient has been symptom-free for several hours, this is a reassuring sign.
- Ask about urine output and the colour of the urine; a reduced or concentrated urine output is suggestive of dehydration.
- Ask about sinister features such as bile in vomitus or blood in stool, as this alludes to an alternative aetiology.

In all but seriously unwell patients, telephone consultations will suffice. Video consultations will help in identifying sunken eyes, dry mucous membranes and skin turgor.

A face-to-face assessment should be considered for patients who are seriously unwell or at risk of becoming dehydrated.

Assessment

- Assess for features of dehydration (see below).
- Perform a urinalysis to assess for ketonuria (indicative of starvation).
- Abdominal tenderness and guarding may be present but will usually be mild.
- Always check blood glucose levels as hypoglycaemia may be a complication, especially in children.

Management

- The mainstay of treatment is hydration and maintaining adequate glucose levels (oral rehydration salts, sugary fluids, ice lollies).

- Other agents which may help with symptom control are analgesics (paracetamol), anti-spasmodics for GI cramps (hyoscine butylbromide 10–20mg QDS × 5 days) and anti-emetics (cyclizine 50mg TDS × 5 days).
- Admission to hospital should be considered if the patient is systemically unwell, dehydrated (dry mucous membranes, tachycardia, hypotension, ketones in the urine) or at risk of dehydration.
- Patients should be referred to their own GP for persistent diarrhoea (over 7 days) or dysentery, as these features warrant a stool sample being sent off for further investigations.

Clinical features of dehydration

Thirst	Decreased skin turgor
Passing less urine	Hypotension
Weight loss	Postural hypotension
Capillary refill time >2s	Tachycardia
Dry mucous membranes	Weak pulses
Sunken eyes	Lethargy

Constipation

Presentation

- This is very much a self-diagnosed condition and although there are standardised tools such as the Bristol stool scale, patients will be unaware of this and constipation will mean different things to different people.
- The patient may not have opened their bowels for several days or may complain of hard stool with pain on passing.
- There will be associated abdominal pain (usually cramping in nature), hard stool, tenesmus, and straining on defecation.
- Complications may include an anal fissure or haemorrhoids, or both.

A face-to-face assessment is rarely required as the diagnosis will be obvious from the patient's history; in most cases patients can be referred to their pharmacist for over-the-counter treatment as well as being given dietary advice and being signposted to appropriate online resources.

Assessment

- Clinical observations will be within normal range.
- Abdominal examination may reveal palpable stool in the left iliac fossa.
- Rectal examination revealing hard stool within the rectum will confirm the diagnosis and assist in ruling out bowel obstruction.

Management

- Most aperients are available over the counter from any pharmacy and these include lactulose (stool softener), ispaghula husk (bulking agent), sennosides (stimulant) and macrogol (osmotic agent).
- Occasionally glycerol suppositories and sodium enemas (e.g. Microlax) may be required, and it can be helpful having these ready when performing a rectal examination.
- If the patient is clinically unwell, in severe pain, vomiting, or if the above measures fail to resolve the constipation, then an admission to hospital for manual evacuation may be required.

Bowel obstruction

Presentation

- Bowel obstruction is characterised by four features: obstipation (unable to pass stool or gas), abdominal distension, abdominal pain and vomiting[1].
- All of these features may not be present during the initial onset, or if the patient has subacute bowel obstruction.
- The patient may have risk factors for bowel obstruction including cancer (30% of colorectal cancers present in an emergency setting[1]), herniae which may be strangulated (tense, tender, negative cough impulse, irreducible), previous abdominal surgery or a previous history of bowel obstruction.

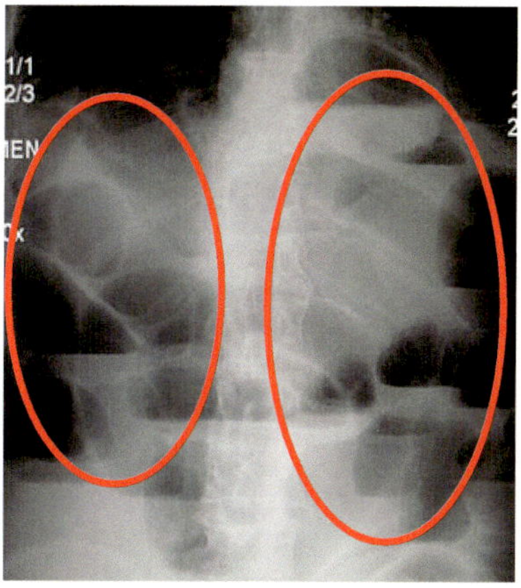

Fig. 11.1: Erect abdominal X-ray demonstrating dilated small bowel loops indicative of small bowel obstruction. A CT scan will confirm the diagnosis.

Patients with obvious bowel obstruction should be referred to ED, as imaging investigations will be required to confirm the diagnosis. In patients where the diagnosis is unclear, a face-to-face assessment is recommended.

Presentation

- Clinical examination will depend on the duration of symptoms.
- Prolonged bowel obstruction can lead to hypovolaemia and haemodynamic shock.
- On examination the abdomen will be distended, tense, tympanic on percussion and tender.

- Bowel sounds may be absent and importantly, the rectum will be empty, helping to differentiate bowel obstruction from severe constipation.

Management

- Patients with suspected bowel obstruction should be referred to the on-call surgeons; although erect abdominal X-rays will demonstrate dilated bowel loops (*Fig. 11.1*), a CT scan of the abdomen will confirm the diagnosis.
- Management is focused on resting the bowels (nil by mouth), fluid resuscitation and treating the underlying cause such as a strangulated hernia.

The four features of bowel obstruction

- Abdominal pain
- Abdominal distension
- Vomiting
- Obstipation

A CT scan of the abdomen will confirm the diagnosis of bowel obstruction.

Gastritis and dyspepsia (indigestion)

Presentation

- Characteristically the patient will have epigastric discomfort, bloating and belching.
- Symptoms will usually be related to food intake.
- Occasionally patients may present with chest pain; however, onset tends to be gradual and the pain will be described more as a burning sensation, as opposed to the central crushing chest pain associated with acute coronary syndrome.
- Features such as diaphoresis, palpitations and shortness of breath are rare and indicate another cause.
- Predisposing risk factors will invariably be present and these include smoking, alcohol, a liking for spicy or fatty foods, NSAID or oral corticosteroid ingestion.
- Psychological and emotional stresses are also significant contributing factors.

Often the diagnosis will be apparent from the history; a video consultation will assist in determining if the patient is in pain and unwell. A face-to-face consultation will be required if the patient is systemically unwell or has atypical features, or if the diagnosis is unclear.

Assessment

- Clinical observations will be within normal limits, as will cardiovascular and respiratory examinations.
- The patient may have tenderness over the epigastrium but guarding and rebound tenderness are rare, and if present point to another diagnosis such as acute pancreatitis.

Management

- Patients who are relatively well can be reassured and advised to reduce or manage risk factors. PPIs (e.g. esomeprazole 20mg OD × 7 days) are available over the counter. H_2 receptor antagonists(20–40mg OD × 7 days) are an alternative, as are alginates (e.g. Gaviscon) which can alleviate the symptoms of gastritis and associated GORD.
- Patients with persistent dyspepsia symptoms may require *H. pylori* investigations, and if results are positive, then eradication treatment will be required.
- Red flag features include haematemesis, melaena, vomiting, symptoms unresponsive to medication, anorexia and weight loss, and observations outside normal range without a clear explanation.
- If these are present the patient should be referred to the on-call gastroenterologists or ED.

Red flag features associated with gastritis

- Haematemesis
- Melaena
- Vomiting
- Anorexia
- Weight loss
- Symptoms unresponsive to medication
- Observations outside normal range without a clear explanation

Acute pancreatitis

Presentation

- Often the presentation will be similar to patients presenting with gastritis; however, the discerning feature is that these patients will be generally unwell.
- There may be a history of gallstones, excessive alcohol consumption or a previous history of acute pancreatitis.

Patients with suspected acute pancreatitis should be assessed face-to-face; however, on some occasions the patient may have had pancreatitis before and be confident that the pain is due to a recurrence. In such cases a video consultation will assist in determining if the patient is severely unwell. If this is the case then an ambulance should be dispatched and immediate transfer to hospital arranged.

Assessment [3]

- The patient may be very unwell, with pallor, diaphoresis, tachycardia and hypotension.
- There will be tenderness and guarding over the epigastric area.
- Rebound tenderness will invariably be present.

Management

- A raised serum amylase confirms the diagnosis; imaging of the pancreas will also help establish the diagnosis.
- Patients with suspected pancreatitis should be referred to the on-call general surgeons or ED so that relevant investigations can be arranged as soon as possible, as acute pancreatitis can be a life-threatening condition.

Differences between acute gastritis and acute pancreatitis

Acute gastritis	vs.	*Acute pancreatitis*
Burning sensation or discomfort		Epigastric pain
Belching		Sweating
Bloating		Vomiting
Normal observations		Abnormal observations
Abdominal examination may be normal		Tender abdomen with guarding
Normal serum amylase		Raised serum amylase

Biliary colic

Presentation[4]

- At the time of presentation the patient may already have been diagnosed with gallstones and may be awaiting a cholecystectomy.
- Characteristically the pain will originate from the right upper quadrant of the abdomen. It will be colicky in nature, often described as coming in waves. Onset will typically be a few hours after food, usually after a meal that is rich in fat.
- The pain may radiate to the right shoulder blade. The four Fs: 'female, fat, fair and forties' do not always apply to patient demographics but are more common in those who present with biliary colic.

Patients with biliary colic will be systemically well and the main symptom will be pain. This can be managed with adequate analgesia which is available over the counter. However, if this is not possible or complications are suspected then the patient should be brought in for a face-to-face assessment.

Assessment

- Importantly, clinical observations are within normal range and there is no overt tenderness of the abdomen.

Management[5]

- This is based on reassurance, fluids, a light diet and analgesia (paracetamol, codeine, NSAIDs). Patients should be referred to their own GP for follow-up and if the diagnosis has not been confirmed, they may require an ultrasound scan to do so.

- The presence of gallstones should be viewed in the context of symptoms, as gallstones do not always cause pain and can often be an incidental finding on ultrasound examination.

Features suggestive of acute cholecystitis and acute hepatitis are:
- Generally unwell patients (e.g. pyrexia, tachycardia).
- Tenderness over the right upper quadrant.
- A positive Murphy's sign (inspiration causes right upper quadrant pain during palpation of the gall bladder).
- Jaundice.

These patients should be referred to the on-call surgical or medical team.

Differences between biliary colic and acute cholecystitis

Biliary colic	vs.	*Acute cholecystitis*
Apyrexial		Pyrexia
Normal pulse rate		Tachycardia
Normal blood pressure		Possible hypotension
Anicteric		Icterus
Abdominal tenderness		Tender abdomen with guarding
Negative Murphy's sign		Positive Murphy's sign

Diverticular disease

Presentation [1]
- With increasing age, diverticulae will increase in number, but they do not always cause symptoms. Complications are inflammation (diverticulitis), bleeding and perforation.
- Diverticulitis will usually present with left iliac fossa pain of insidious onset and patients will usually be over 50 years of age.

Patients who are systemically well can be assessed over the phone and via video consultation; often patients can point to the area of pain and will be able to self-palpate the area and elicit tenderness.

In all other cases and especially in the elderly, consider a face-to-face assessment, as the risk of complications as well as the possibility of an alternative diagnosis such as a leaking aneurysm is higher.

Assessment
- Depending on the nature and severity of complications the patient may be pyrexic and tachycardic.
- On palpation of the abdomen there will be tenderness, with guarding over the affected area.

- A rectal examination will be normal unless there is bleeding within the bowel, in which case haematochezia will be present.

Management[6]

- This is centred on pain relief (avoid opiates as these can cause constipation), laxatives (bulking agents are preferred) and antibiotics (as bacterial overgrowth within the diverticulae is considered to be a contributing factor to diverticulitis).
- Co-amoxiclav 625mg PO TDS × 5 days or cephalexin 500mg PO TDS with metronidazole 400mg PO TDS × 5 days are usually prescribed.
- If there is bleeding or suspicion of a perforation (shock, peritonitis), the patient should be transferred to hospital immediately.

Irritable bowel syndrome (IBS)

Presentation

- This is a very common condition.
- It is a chronic condition often following a relapsing–remitting course, but without any life-threatening sequelae. Symptoms occur due to GI dysmotility related to smooth muscle or nerve dysfunction within the GI tract.
- Often patients will have an established diagnosis or present with an acute exacerbation of long-standing symptoms.
- Several triggers have been implicated, including certain foods, emotional and psychological stress and post GI infections.
- Common presenting symptoms include bloating, abdominal cramps, alternating diarrhoea and constipation, flatulence and tenesmus.

Most patients can be assessed over the phone; the chronicity of the condition and the presence of long-standing symptoms without progression are reassuring factors (although maybe not for the patient). Patients may also have had investigations in the past which were reported as being normal. Medication to manage symptoms is usually available over the counter and a face-to-face assessment is rarely required unless there are red flag features such as rectal bleeding or weight loss, as these would suggest alternative pathology.

Assessment

- Patients will look well and general observations will be in normal range.
- Abdominal examination will be normal.

Management

- This is a lifelong condition with no 'cure'.
- It is important to address underlying emotional and psychological stresses as well as anxiety.
- Dietary modification will also help, although the changes required will vary per patient. There is no specific diet which will help all patients.
- Anti-spasmodic agents such as mebeverine, alverine and hyoscine butylbromide (Buscopan) will help with cramps.

- Peppermint oil capsules will help with bloating.
- Aperients can be used to manage predominantly constipation symptoms; loperamide can be used to manage predominantly diarrhoea symptoms.
- Amitriptyline can also help and is believed to have analgesic and neuromodulatory benefits.
- Patients should be advised to follow up with their own GP to discuss long-term management options.

Ano-rectal conditions

Haemorrhoids

- Can be asymptomatic.
- Common presenting features tend to be pain, a palpable lump and bright red rectal bleeding, often filling the whole toilet pan.
- Patients may volunteer a history of straining or hard stool.
- A healthy diet full of fibre, and topical ointments (e.g. Anusol or Proctosedyl), which are available from the pharmacy, will help to alleviate symptoms.
- Internal haemorrhoids can be managed with suppositories, which are also available from the pharmacy (e.g. Anusol suppositories).

Anal fissures

- These will present with pain and occasional bleeding.
- The pain can be intense and spasmodic.
- Rectal examination will be intensely painful and often impossible.
- Management is focused on a healthy diet with plenty of fibre, stool softeners (e.g. lactulose), and topical agents (e.g. GTN ointment or diltiazem cream) can help with sphincter spasm and healing.

Perianal abscesses

- These will be extremely painful.
- Patients will be able to locate the exact origin and due to the recurrent nature may volunteer the diagnosis.
- A general examination is essential to rule out sepsis.
- Antibiotics will only be of benefit if the infection and abscess has not become established.
- A common regime is amoxicillin 500mg TDS with metronidazole 400mg TDS × 7 days.
- Once an abscess has arisen the only option will be incision and drainage. In such cases, or if the patient is systemically unwell, a referral to the on-call surgeons is warranted.

Summary for gastroenterology

- The 'Hamburger test' is 80% sensitive for anorexia.
- Acute appendicitis can present with vague symptoms and signs, especially in patients who present early through the course of their symptoms.
- The four features of bowel obstruction are obstipation (inability to pass stool or gas), abdominal distension, abdominal pain and vomiting. All of these may not be evident in all patients at the time of presentation.
- Consider referred pain from inguinal or femoral herniae, as well as testicular pathology in men.
- Signs of peritonitis are tenderness, guarding and rebound tenderness. The presence of these features is an indication for referral to hospital.
- Red flag features of dyspepsia include haematemesis, melaena, vomiting, symptoms unresponsive to medication, weight and appetite loss, and observations outside normal range without a clear explanation.

References

1. The Royal College of Surgeons of England (2014) *Commissioning Guide: Emergency general surgery (acute abdominal pain)*. Available at: www.rcseng.ac.uk/library-and-publications/rcs-publications/docs/emergency-general-guide/

2. de Virgilio, C., Frank, P.N. and Grigorian, A. (2015) *Surgery: a case based clinical review*. Springer, p. 215.

3. NICE (updated 2020) *Pancreatitis* [NG104]. Available at: www.nice.org.uk/guidance/ng104

4. NICE (2014) *Gallstone disease: diagnosis and management* [CG188]. Available at: www.nice.org.uk/guidance/cg188

5. The Royal College of Surgeons of England (2013) *Gallstones – Commissioning Guide*. Available at: www.rcseng.ac.uk/library-and-publications/rcs-publications/docs/gallstones-commissioning-guide/

6. NICE (revised 2023) *Diverticular disease management*. Available at: https://cks.nice.org.uk/diverticular-disease

12

Chapter 12: **Rheumatology**

"Life without limbs? Or life without limits?"
Nick Vujicic

Assessment of patients presenting with rheumatological problems

Telephone

- A detailed history can be taken over the phone.
- Enquire about medical problems, medication and predisposers to serious conditions.
- Often patients may have had a recurrence of a condition and it is important to enquire about this and how it was managed in the past.
- Images and video consultations may help in certain conditions (e.g. gout).
- Video consultations can help in ascertaining range of movement at joints as well as any skin changes; however, in most cases a face-to-face assessment will be required to assess the affected part of the body.
- The presence of acute headaches in the elderly should be considered a red flag symptom; more so if there are visual disturbances as this is suggestive of temporal or giant cell arteritis, which requires immediate intervention.

Face-to-face

- Have a low threshold for face-to-face assessments for the elderly.
- If there are systemic features (e.g. pyrexia) consider a face-to-face assessment.
- Assess and document general observations.

Temporal (giant cell) arteritis

Presentation[1]

- This is a vasculitis where there is granulomatous inflammation of medium- to large-sized arteries.
- It is uncommon in patients less than 55 years of age.
- There may be a history of polymyalgia rheumatica (in 50% of those affected) or previous visual disturbances.
- Characteristically there will be pain over the temporal areas.

Patients who are suspected of having temporal arteritis should be assessed face-to-face.

Assessment

- Observations will be within normal range.
- The condition is characterised by dilated, palpable and tender arteries over the temporal areas (*Fig 12.1*).
- Visual disturbances such as double vision or complete loss of vision may affect one or both eyes; hence consider assessing visual fields and performing fundoscopy.

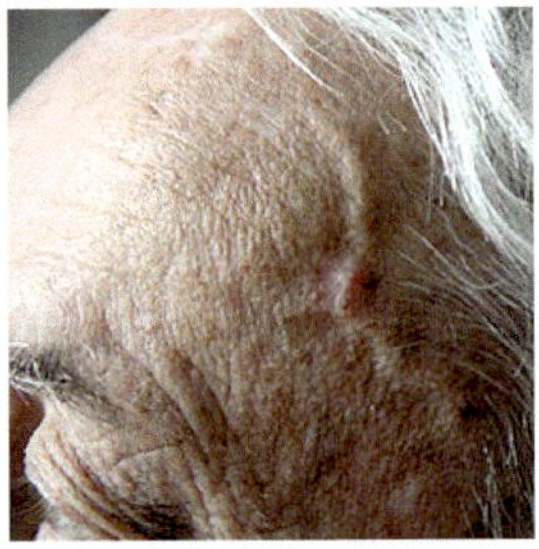

Fig. 12.1: Superficial temporal artery – becomes firm and tender in temporal arteritis.

Management[2]

- This is a medical emergency and untreated temporal arteritis can cause blindness, so early diagnosis and treatment is essential.
- Patients should have blood tests for inflammatory markers such as ESR and CRP. Elevated levels support the diagnosis of temporal arteritis.
- Temporal artery biopsy will not always be diagnostic due to the presence of skip lesions, and therefore treatment should not be delayed if temporal arteritis is suspected.
- If temporal arteritis is suspected, start prednisolone 60mg and refer the patient to the on-call medical team.
- Also consider adding in aspirin 75mg OD with a PPI such as lansoprazole 15mg OD.

Bursitis

Presentation

- Bursae are small fluid-filled sacs that overlie bony prominences; notably the elbow, knee, shoulder, heel and hip.
- Bursitis occurs when a bursa becomes inflamed; this can occur due to repetitive trauma or an infection.
- The bursa will be swollen, erythematous, warm, painful and tender.

Although the diagnosis can be suspected over the phone, often a visual assessment may be required. This can be done via video consultation or in person.

Assessment

- Patients will be systemically well and observations will be in normal range, unless the bursa is infected. In this case the patient may have a temperature and associated tachycardia.
- The affected bursa will be swollen, warm, tender and fluctuant.
- It is important to assess the joint underneath the bursa as there is a risk that infection may spread and involve the joint, resulting in septic arthritis (see below).

Management
- Avoid any precipitating factors such as trauma or friction to the area.
- Apply ice to reduce swelling.
- An elasticated bandage will help to manage the swelling.
- Oral NSAIDs such as ibuprofen or naproxen will help to alleviate pain and inflammation.
- If an infection is suspected then antibiotics can be prescribed, with flucloxacillin 500mg QDS × 7 days being first-line and clarithromycin 500mg BD × 7 days for those who are allergic to penicillin. Often several weeks of antibiotics may be required.
- Diagnostic and therapeutic aspiration should only be undertaken by a qualified clinician and in an aseptic environment.
- The presence of systemic symptoms or failure to respond to antibiotics warrants a referral to the on-call orthopaedic surgeons.

Gout

Presentation
- Gout is characterised by raised uric acid levels in the serum, resulting in urate crystals being deposited in a joint, which then results in acute inflammation.
- Gout has a higher incidence in males, although post-menopausal females are just as likely to be affected as men.
- Common contributory factors are foods (red meat, offal and seafood), alcohol, thiazide diuretics, medical conditions (diabetes mellitus, haematological malignancies) and a family history.
- Presentations seem to peak after a holiday in the sun or after an over-indulgent festive season.
- Patients may present with a recurrence so enquire about how previous episodes were managed.

Often the diagnosis is apparent on the phone; a video consultation may help in confirming the diagnosis. If there is any doubt a face-to-face assessment should be arranged.

Assessment
- The affected joint is painful, erythematous (*Fig. 12.2*), warm and exquisitely tender.
- The absence of trauma to the joint increases the likelihood of the prime suspect being gout.
- It can occur in any joint; however, the most commonly affected joint is the 1st metatarsophalangeal joint (MTPJ) of the foot.
- It is important to exclude septic arthritis as a potential cause of symptoms, and a normal temperature, pulse and blood pressure can assist in doing this.

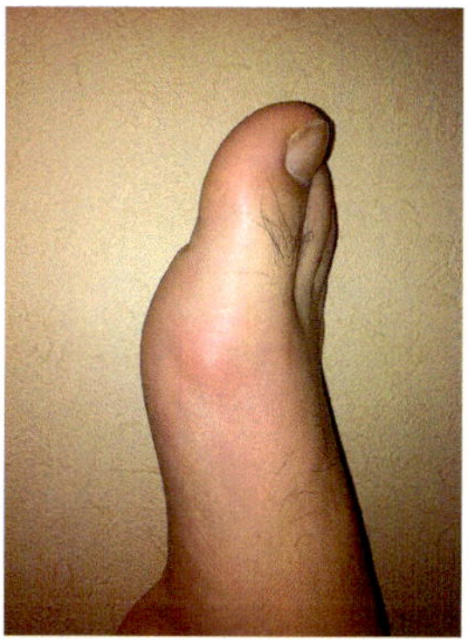

Fig. 12.2: Gouty inflammation of the 1st MTPJ.

Management[3]

- Treatment is primarily with NSAIDs such as ibuprofen 400mg TDS × 7 days (bear in mind this may not be strong enough) or naproxen 250mg QDS × 7 days. Consider prescribing or asking the patient to purchase a PPI from the pharmacy to protect against the side-effects of NSAIDs.
- An alternative is colchicine 500mcg BD; this is titrated up until pain relief is achieved or adverse effects are intolerable.
- Oral prednisolone 30mg OD × 5 days can be prescribed to patients who cannot take NSAIDs and are unable to tolerate colchicine[4].
- In addition to medication patients should be encouraged to drink plenty of fluids (non-alcoholic) and address dietary and other risk factors.
- If there is doubt between the diagnosis of gout and septic arthritis the patient should be referred to the on-call orthopaedic surgeons for further investigations.
- Patients with two or more episodes of gout should be advised to speak to their GP to discuss prophylactic treatment and to prevent irreversible damage to the affected joints.

Septic arthritis

Presentation

- This can affect any joint, and presents with an insidious onset of pain, swelling and erythema.
- The absence of trauma or a sprain should raise suspicions of septic arthritis.
- There may also be predisposing factors such as diabetes mellitus, an overlying skin condition or an overlying wound.

Although a video consultation may assist in ascertaining the diagnosis, a face-to-face assessment is recommended to confirm the diagnosis and to determine the severity, as well as assessing for features of systemic upset.

Assessment[5],[6]

- Patients may be generally unwell, with a high temperature and tachycardia helping to differentiate it from gout.
- The affected joint will be very painful, warm and exquisitely tender, with a restricted and painful range of movement (often passive and active movement will be completely absent).
- A raised white cell count and CRP will be evident on blood investigations.
- Diagnostic arthrocentesis should only be undertaken within aseptic conditions and in a hospital setting.

Management

- Patients with suspected septic arthritis should be referred to the on call orthopaedic team.
- A delay in assessment and treatment can result in irreversible damage to the affected joint.

Differences between gout and septic arthritis

Gout	vs.	*Septic arthritis*
More common in men		Just as common in women
Middle-aged		Older person
Dietary risk factors		No dietary risk factors
Linked to medication, e.g. thiazides		May be on immunosuppressants
Relatively sudden onset		Gradual onset
Normal temperature		Low-grade pyrexia
Normal heart rate		Tachycardia
Small joints affected, e.g. MTPJ		Larger joint affected, e.g. knee
No overlying injury		Possible penetrating skin injury
Some joint mobility		Almost complete loss of mobility
Oral NSAIDs or colchicine		Refer to hospital

Acute (on chronic) osteoarthritis

Presentation

- Patients will usually be elderly with a pre-existing history of osteoarthritis.
- There may be a trigger such as a sprain or overuse preceding presentation.

This can be difficult to differentiate from septic arthritis or an inflammatory arthritis over the phone. Therefore unless there is a history of a previous occurrence of acute on chronic osteoarthritis with similar presenting features, a face-to-face assessment is recommended.

Assessment and management

- General observations will be within normal range.
- The aggravated joint will be painful and swollen, with clinical evidence of degeneration.
- Usually the overlying skin will be of normal temperature and will be normal in colour.
- The range of movement will be limited, but not to the degree associated with a septic joint.
- Assessment should focus on ruling out septic arthritis, with the mainstay of treatment being pain relief and gentle mobilisation once symptoms abate.
- The patient should be advised to follow up with their own GP to discuss management options.

Inflammatory arthritides

Presentation

- The patient may already have an established diagnosis of an inflammatory arthropathy such as rheumatoid arthritis.
- Patients may also be on long-term treatment such as methotrexate.

- Exacerbations may affect one joint or result in generalised arthralgia affecting the whole body.

A face-to-face assessment is rarely required as most patients will and should have a plan in place for acute exacerbations. Often the reason for the contact will be to obtain a prescription for a short supply of medication to bring the exacerbation under control.

Assessment

- A generalised stiffness may be reported and demonstrated.
- General observations will be within normal range.

Management

- This is centred on pain relief and releasing the inflammatory restraints.
- This is done with oral NSAIDs or oral prednisolone 20mg once daily × 5 days[4].
- Occasionally intramuscular corticosteroids may be required, such as methylprednisolone 40mg IM stat[7].

Summary for rheumatology

- A painful joint in the absence of an injury should raise suspicions of gout or septic arthritis.
- The presence of a high temperature and tachycardia can assist in differentiating septic arthritis from gout.
- Think temporal (giant cell) arteritis in elderly patients who present with an acute headache and visual disturbances.

References

1. Vasculitis UK (no date) *What is giant cell arteritis / temporal arteritis?* Available at: www.vasculitis.org.uk/about-vasculitis/giant-cell-arteritis-temporal-arteritis

2. NICE (revised 2024) *Management of giant cell arteritis*. Available at: https://cks.nice.org.uk/topics/giant-cell-arteritis/management/management/

3. Hui, M., Carr, A., Cameron, S. *et al.*, for the British Society for Rheumatology Standards, Audit and Guidelines Working Group (2017) The British Society for Rheumatology guideline for the management of gout. *Rheumatology*, **56(7):** e1–e20. Available at: https://doi.org/10.1093/rheumatology/kex156

4. BNF (no date) *Prednisolone*. Available at: https://bnf.nice.org.uk/drug/prednisolone.html

5. Coakley, G. and Mathews, C.J. (2020) Septic arthritis. *BMJ Best Practice*. Available at: https://bestpractice.bmj.com/topics/en-gb/486

6. Visser, S. and Tupper, J. (2009) Septic until proven otherwise: approach to and treatment of the septic joint in adult patients. *Can Fam Physician*, **55(4):** 374–375.

7. BNF (no date) *Methylprednisolone*. Available at: https://bnf.nice.org.uk/drug/methylprednisolone.html#indicationsAndDoses

13

Chapter 13: **Urology**

"What lies behind us and what lies before us are tiny matters compared to what lies within us."
Ralph Waldo Emerson

Assessment of patients with acute urological conditions

Telephone

- A detailed history can be taken over the phone.
- Some patients may have access to diagnostic equipment such as a thermometer or an automated sphygmomanometer at home; these can be really helpful when trying to decide if a patient with a urinary tract infection (UTI) may have sepsis.
- A video consultation may also assist in determining if a patient is acutely unwell.

Face-to-face

Face-to-face assessment would be required in the following situations:

- The patient has systemic symptoms.
- The patient has prolonged symptoms.
- The patient is at high risk of developing complications, e.g. immunocompromised and has a suspected UTI.
- There is diagnostic uncertainty.

Cystitis

Presentation

- Cystitis refers to inflammation of the bladder, and this is not always due to an infection.
- Although more common in women, it can also occur in men.
- Symptoms include dysuria, frequency of micturition, hesitancy of micturition, suprapubic pain or discomfort, and cloudy urine.
- The patient will be systemically well.

In most cases the diagnosis can be made over the phone – patients can be signposted to their pharmacy for over-the-counter treatment as well as appropriate online resources.

A face-to-face assessment is very rarely required, unless it is suspected there is an alternative cause for the patient's symptoms.

Assessment

- General observations will be within normal range.

- Abdominal examination tends to be normal, although some patients may have some suprapubic tenderness.
- Urine dipstick is usually (but not always) positive for leucocytes and blood.
- The presence of nitrates (by-product of bacteria metabolism) indicates bacteriuria.

Management

- Not all patients will require antibiotics. Most cases will resolve spontaneously; paracetamol and ibuprofen and plenty of fluids will help[1].
- Oral potassium citrate or sodium bicarbonate solutions (available from the pharmacy) are believed to reduce the acidity of the urine and assist in alleviating symptoms; however, the evidence for their efficacy is limited, as is the case with cranberry juice and D-mannose.
- A delayed prescription for antibiotics, with instructions to start them if symptoms do not resolve in 48 hours, may help reassure patients and treat persistent symptoms due to a subacute infection which will not clear with conservative measures.

Urinary tract infections

Presentation

- UTIs are more common in women.
- Symptoms are very similar to those in patients presenting with cystitis; however, patients may have systemic features such as a high temperature and tachycardia.
- Simple UTIs in patients who do not have any underlying conditions can be managed by their community pharmacist, and therefore patients can be referred to their local pharmacy.
- Often UTIs may be recurrent and the patient will be able to self-diagnose the condition.

If the patient is systemically well, has had antibiotics in the past for a UTI and there is appropriate safety-netting in place, then a prescription can be issued via telephone triage.

Patients can also present to their local pharmacy, as most pharmacies now offer a urinalysis service and if an infection is confirmed, the pharmacist is able to dispense a course of antibiotics.

A face-to-face assessment may be required for patients where the diagnosis is uncertain, the patient is generally unwell or is at risk of developing complications.

Assessment

- A general examination including observations is essential to rule out sepsis.
- Abdominal examination should be undertaken to rule out urinary retention and other causes of abdominal pain.
- Flank or loin tenderness may be present if the infection has ascended to involve the kidneys.
- Observations and examination findings (both positive and negative) should be recorded in the contemporaneous notes.

- The urine dipstick will reveal blood and leucocytes indicative of inflammation within the renal tract; the presence of nitrates will confirm bacteriuria.

Management[2],[3]

- Conservative measures such as drinking plenty of fluids and oral analgesia will help.
- Commonly prescribed antibiotics are trimethoprim 200mg BD or nitrofurantoin MR (modified release) 100mg BD, or pivmecillinam 400mg stat then 200mg TDS × 3 days or co-amoxiclav 625mg TDS (usually reserved for complicated UTIs).
- Three days of antibiotics are usually enough for uncomplicated UTIs.
- Men who present with frequent UTIs should be investigated for underlying conditions and the possibility of sexually transmitted infections which can present with similar symptoms to a UTI.
- Seven days of antibiotics may be required in patients with a complicated UTI (systemically unwell, haematuria), in men, or in patients with indwelling urethral catheters.

UTIs in pregnancy

- Pregnant women with a suspected UTI should always be treated due to the increased risk of miscarriage and premature labour.
- If there is a high index of suspicion, antibiotics can be started whilst culture results are awaited. Antibiotics which can be prescribed are nitrofurantoin in the first 24 weeks of pregnancy or trimethoprim after the first 12 weeks of pregnancy.
- Amoxicillin and cephalexin are alternatives.

Asymptomatic bacteriuria

- This is common in the elderly and those who have indwelling urethral catheters.
- Asymptomatic patients who have nitrates only on urine dipstick or microorganism-positive urine cultures without symptoms do not require treatment.

Important notes

- When assessing patients with a UTI, sepsis must be ruled out.
- UTIs in pregnancy must be treated due to the increased risk of miscarriage.
- Men who present with severe or recurrent UTIs should be investigated for underlying pathology.
- Asymptomatic bacteriuria is common in the elderly and does not require treatment.

Pyelonephritis

Presentation

- Pyelonephritis refers to infection of the renal pelvis, i.e. upper urinary tract.
- The source of the infection can be either ascending, from the bladder or via the bloodstream.

- There may be a history of predisposing conditions such as diabetes mellitus, chronic kidney disease and immunocompromise.
- Patients will express symptoms of a UTI but will also have systemic symptoms such as malaise, nausea, vomiting and pyrexia.

It is recommended that all patients with suspected pyelonephritis have a face-to-face assessment due to the high risk of complications and sepsis.

Features of pyelonephritis

- Frank pyuria
- Flank tenderness
- Pyrexia
- Tachycardia
- Hypotension

Assessment

- The patient will look unwell, with pallor and diaphoresis.
- Patients with pyelonephritis will be systemically unwell and there may be features suggestive of sepsis, such as tachycardia, hypotension and pyrexia.
- There will be loin or flank tenderness with frank pyuria (pus in the urine).

Management[4]

- Although mild cases can be managed in the community with oral antibiotics (e.g. cephalexin 500mg BD or co-amoxiclav 625mg TDS for 7 days) there should be an extremely low threshold for referral to hospital, as complications such as sepsis can manifest at an alarming pace.
- Appropriate safety-netting is mandatory, and consider a follow-up telephone call in 48 hours to reassess the patient.

Renal colic

The most common cause of renal or ureteric colic is a calculus (stone).

Presentation

- Patients with renal colic will be in severe pain radiating from the loin to the groin.
- The pain will be of sudden onset and colicky in nature.
- Commonly associated features include nausea, vomiting, dysuria and frank haematuria.
- There may be a previous history of renal calculi.
- Predisposing factors include hypercalcaemia, dehydration, metabolic disorders or a family history.

A video consultation may help to determine the severity of the pain the patient is in and whether a direct referral to ED is warranted, as often a CT KUB will be required within 24 hours to confirm the diagnosis and to identify complications such as hydronephrosis.

Assessment

- Observations will be normal unless the patient is in severe pain or has a concomitant UTI.
- Urine dipstick will reveal blood, and occasionally leucocytes.
- The presence of nitrates confirms bacteriuria and suggests a concomitant UTI.

Management[5]

- This is centred on pain relief, with NSAIDs (e.g. diclofenac) being first-line agents; these can be administered orally or rectally.
- Alternatives or adjuncts include paracetamol 1g QDS or co-codamol 30/500 mg two tablets QDS.
- Tamsulosin 400mcg OD can be used to alleviate ureter spasm.
- All patients will require a CT KUB or ultrasound within 24 hours to rule out hydronephrosis and kidney injury.
- If the pain is severe or there is frank haematuria or suspected hydronephrosis, the patient should be referred to ED or the on-call urology team.

A CT KUB should be requested within 24 hours of presentation of a patient with suspected renal calculi. It is the investigation of choice to confirm renal calculi and rule out hydronephrosis.

Acute urinary retention

Presentation

- This requires immediate medical attention; onset tends to be over a few hours.
- The patient will volunteer the diagnosis and be in discomfort or even pain.
- There can be various causes including prostate hypertrophy, prostate cancer, constipation, UTIs, and medication (e.g. tricyclic antidepressants), or it can be idiopathic.

A face-to-face assessment should be undertaken where a bladder scanner is available and there are facilities to catheterise. If this is not possible the patient should be referred directly to the ED.

Assessment

- There will be a palpable bladder, felt as a mass arising from the pelvis.
- On applying gentle suprapubic pressure the patient will feel the urge to micturate.
- A bladder scan will confirm the diagnosis.

Management

- Urethral catheterisation is vital to allow the bladder to empty and relieve pressure within the urinary tract.
- Catheterisation should be undertaken in a sterile environment and by a trained clinician with appropriate equipment.
- If this is not available the patient should be referred to ED or the on-call urology team.

Summary for urology

- Cystitis refers to inflammation of the bladder and is not always due to a UTI.
- Mild UTIs can clear with conservative measures; however, consider issuing a delayed prescription with appropriate advice.
- Patients with all but mild pyelonephritis should be referred to hospital.
- Patients with suspected renal colic should have a CT KUB within 24 hours to rule out hydronephrosis or an acute kidney injury.

References

1. NHS (no date) *Overview: Cystitis*. Available at: www.nhs.uk/conditions/cystitis/

2. NICE (2018) *Urinary tract infection (lower): antimicrobial prescribing* [NG109]. Available at: www.nice.org.uk/guidance/ng109

3. NICE (no date) *Urinary-tract infections*. Available at: https://bnf.nice.org.uk/treatment-summary/urinary-tract-infections.html

4. NICE (revised 2024) *Pyelonephritis – acute*. Available at: https://cks.nice.org.uk/pyelonephritis-acute#!scenario

5. NICE (2019) *Renal and ureteric stones: assessment and management* [NG118]. Available at: www.nice.org.uk/guidance/ng118/chapter/Recommendations

14

Chapter 14: **Ophthalmology**

"Few are those who see with their own eyes and feel with their own hearts."
Albert Einstein

Assessment of patients presenting with acute eye conditions

Telephone

- The two most important features to consider when assessing acute eye conditions are pain and acuity.
- Eye injuries and foreign bodies will usually require slit lamp assessment with fluorescein dye, and patients should be referred to an appropriate urgent treatment centre.
- Any chemical or thermal injuries to the eye should be referred to ED or the on-call ophthalmology team.
- A detailed history will usually provide a clear indication of whether the patient can be seen in a primary care setting or will require an ED or ophthalmology referral.

Face-to-face

- If there is any doubt with regard to the diagnosis and it is unclear if the patient should be referred directly to hospital, consider a face-to-face assessment.
- An objective assessment of visual acuity using a Snellen chart is required.
- If there is an acute onset of pain or a proven drop in visual acuity (assessed via a Snellen chart) the patient should be referred to ED or the on-call ophthalmology team.
- In addition to assessing visual acuity, a face-to-face assessment should include an assessment of pupil reflexes and of range of movement of the eye.
- If a corneal injury is suspected, a slit lamp examination with fluorescein should also be conducted.

Red flags for ophthalmology

Acute onset of pain or a sudden drop in visual acuity are indications for referral to ED or the on-call ophthalmology team.

Conjunctivitis

Presentation

There are three main types of conjunctivitis.

Often the aetiology can be determined over the phone; if there is any doubt a video consultation and still images should help confirm the diagnosis. A face-to-face consultation is rarely required.

- **Bacterial conjunctivitis**
  - more common in the young
  - presents with a purulent discharge
  - it is a benign and self-limiting condition
  - pain is absent and visual acuity will remain intact
  - occasionally patients may complain of blurred vision; however, this will clear on blinking
  - symptoms settle within 7 days with regular eye bathing (wipe the eye using cotton wool and cooled boiled water four times a day)
  - chloramphenicol 0.5% eye drops (available over the counter) or chloramphenicol 1% ointment applied four times a day can be prescribed and both have been shown to shorten the duration of symptoms[1].
- **Viral conjunctivitis**
  - the eye tends to be watery and red with a gritty sensation
  - it is highly contagious and commonly affects both eyes
  - it is self-limiting and symptoms usually settle within 7 days
  - lubricating eye drops containing hypromellose (available from the pharmacy) can be used to keep the eye comfortable
  - if inflammation of the conjunctiva is marked, topical ketorolac eye drops can be prescribed
  - corticosteroid eye drops should only be initiated by an ophthalmologist due to the risk of sight-threatening complications in the presence of a concomitant viral ulcer of the cornea
  - patients should be advised to avoid sharing towels and to wash hands after touching their eyes, due to the contagious nature of the condition.
- **Allergic conjunctivitis**
  - this commonly affects both eyes
  - it is associated with allergic rhinitis
  - the eyes are watery, red and feel itchy
  - management centres around avoiding the trigger and using oral antihistamines such as chlorphenamine 4mg every 6 hours or cetirizine 10mg once daily
  - sodium cromoglycate eye drops can also help alleviate symptoms; these are available from the pharmacy.

Stye (hordeolum)

Presentation and assessment

- A stye is an infection of one of the hair follicles on the eyelid, and presents as a small painful swelling (*Fig. 14.1*).
- This is different to a chalazion which is a granuloma of the meibomian glands and tends to be a hard painless swelling of the eyelid.

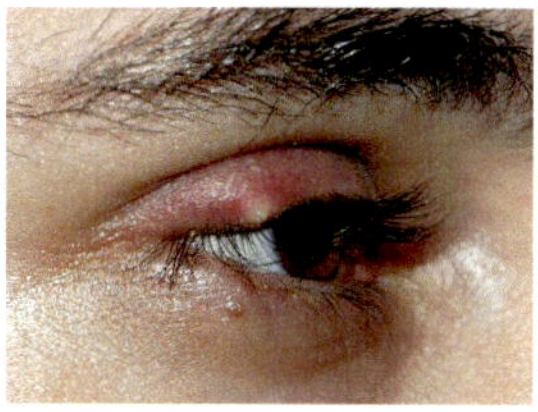

Fig. 14.1: Stye (hordeolum) after approximately 5 days.

Reproduced from https://commons.wikimedia.org/wiki/File:Stye02.jpg Public domain (photo by Andre Riemann).

A face-to-face assessment or video consultation is often required to differentiate a stye from a chalazion and also to ensure there are no signs of periorbital cellulitis.

Management

- In the majority of cases a stye will resolve spontaneously.
- Resolution can be expedited with warm compresses, regular bathing of the eyelid and cleaning the affected area with a cotton bud soaked in a diluted solution of baby shampoo.
- Severely infected styes can be treated with topical chloramphenicol 0.5% eye drops and oral antibiotics such as flucloxacillin 500mg QDS or clarithromycin 500mg BD for 7 days.

Periorbital (preseptal) and orbital cellulitis

Presentation and assessment

Although a detailed history can be taken over the phone, all patients with suspected periorbital or orbital cellulitis should be assessed face-to-face.

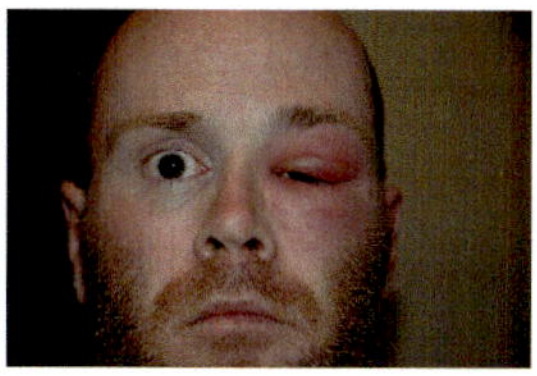

Fig. 14.2: Periorbital (pre-septal) cellulitis.

Reproduced from www.flickr.com/photos/trippchicago/4316733120/ under a CC BY 2.0 licence (photo by Tripp).

It is important to be able to differentiate between the two conditions and also to ensure there are no features of sepsis or systemic upset.

- A general examination to identify signs of systemic infection is mandatory.
- Orbital cellulitis is an ophthalmological emergency.
- Orbital cellulitis can be differentiated from periorbital cellulitis as the pain will be intra-orbital, deep-seated and more severe.
- Patients with orbital cellulitis tend to be systemically unwell.
- Orbital cellulitis will result in reduced visual acuity and a limited range of movement of the globe of the eye (this is not the case with periorbital cellulitis).

Management

- An emergency referral to the on-call ophthalmology team is mandatory if orbital cellulitis is suspected.
- Periorbital cellulitis (*Fig. 14.2*) can be managed with oral antibiotics such as co-amoxiclav; however, if it does not respond to oral antibiotics or the patient is systemically unwell, they should be referred to the on-call medical team.

Subconjunctival haemorrhage

Often the diagnosis can be made on the phone; images and video consultations can also be utilised. Face-to-face consultations may be required if there is suspected trauma to the eye and to ensure blood pressure is within normal range.

Presentation and assessment

- Although it can be an alarming condition for the patient and visually quite striking (*Fig. 14.3*), it is completely benign.
- A subconjunctival haemorrhage will manifest itself quite suddenly.
- It may be spontaneous or it may be brought on by a coughing or a sneezing episode.
- Occasionally there may be a history of minor trauma to the eye.
- Some patients may be on antiplatelet or anticoagulant medication, and this is considered to be a contributory factor.

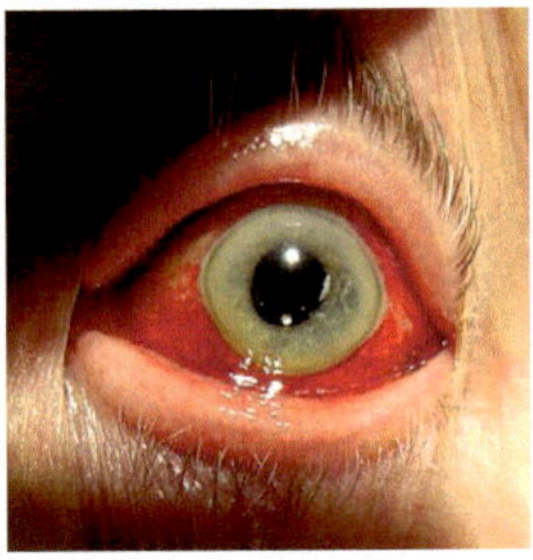

Fig. 14.3: Eye showing subconjunctival haemorrhage.

Management

- This is based on ensuring there are no underlying risk factors such as hypertension (hence it is important to check the blood pressure).
- Reassurance that this is a benign and self-limiting condition.
- Lubricating eye drops (e.g. hypromellose) to alleviate any discomfort.
- Complete resolution should be expected within 2 weeks.

Corneal abrasion

Presentation

- Patients are often able to identify a trigger or the exact time when a foreign body may have caused the injury.
- Discomfort is more common than pain.

- A drop in visual acuity is rare.

A face-to-face assessment is required; nearly always a slit lamp examination and fluorescein dye will be required to delineate the abrasion and rule out corneal ulcers and extract corneal foreign bodies. For these reasons patients with suspected corneal injuries should only be referred to primary care or urgent treatment centres where these facilities are available.

Assessment

- The abrasion can usually be seen using topical fluorescein dye and with a slit lamp or an ophthalmoscope blue light.
- It is important to ensure there are no foreign bodies.
- Always examine behind the upper and lower eyelids.

Management

- Most abrasions heal spontaneously within a few days.
- Chloramphenicol 0.5% eye drops can be prescribed to prevent secondary bacterial infections.

Corneal foreign bodies

- These can be removed by using topical anaesthetic and either cotton wool or the edge of a bevelled needle.
- Topical chloramphenicol eye drops should be prescribed after removal of the foreign body and a reassessment should take place 5 days later to ensure injuries are healing.

Summary for ophthalmology

- A sudden drop in visual acuity or a sudden onset of pain is an indication to refer to the on-call ophthalmologist.
- Chemical or thermal injuries of the eye should be referred to hospital.
- The most common types of conjunctivitis are viral, bacterial and allergic.
- Corneal injuries can be seen with fluorescein and a blue light (slit lamp or ophthalmoscope).
- Patients should be reassessed 5 days after the removal of any foreign bodies from the eye.
- Topical corticosteroid drops for acute eye problems should be initiated by an ophthalmologist.

Reference

1. Jefferis, J., Perera, R., Everitt, H. *et al.* (2011) Acute infective conjunctivitis in primary care: who needs antibiotics? An individual data meta-analysis. *British Journal of General Practice*, **61(590):** e542–e548.

15

Chapter 15: **Mental health**

"Most of us have far more courage than we ever dreamed we possessed."
Dale Carnegie

Assessment of patients who present with acute mental health problems

Telephone

- Most patients who present with a mental health problem can be assessed over the telephone.
- A detailed history can be taken: ask about previous episodes, relapses and compliance with medication.
- Enquire about support the patient may have and who is with the patient during the consultation.
- Consider speaking to family members or friends.
- Patients can be signposted to appropriate resources such as their local pharmacist for over-the-counter medication which may help with their symptoms, e.g. promethazine for insomnia.
- If there is a risk of harm to the patient or others, consider calling the police and paramedics.
- Patients who are suicidal should be referred to ED and the on-call crisis team or psychiatric liaison nurse.
- Video consultations can also help as this will allow a visual assessment of the patient in their surroundings; it will allow you to pick up any features such as psychomotor agitation or retardation.

A face-to-face assessment may be required to rule out a physical cause for the patient's symptoms, for example if a suspected UTI is causing acute confusion.

Acute stress, anxiety and depression

Presentation

- These conditions should ideally be managed by the patient's own GP as they require regular follow-up, counselling and monitoring for any adverse effects medication may cause.
- The majority of patients may already have a diagnosis of a mental health disorder.
- A life event or a culmination of factors may be responsible for the acute presentation.
- It may be possible to reassure patients and to talk them through this stressful period.

- Patients can also be signposted to available resources, including NHS counselling services, occupational health services, websites and phone apps to help manage their condition, as well as being referred to their own GP.

In the majority of cases telephone triage, reassurance, signposting, ensuring adequate support and a follow-up with the patient's own GP will be enough.

On rare occasions it may be necessary to prescribe medication; in such circumstances consider a face-to-face assessment.

Management [1]

- Patients presenting acutely can be prescribed a very short supply of medication (i.e. for 2–3 days) until a review by the patient's own GP can be undertaken.
- It is always a case of weighing up potential pitfalls with benefits when prescribing medication to someone who presents with an acute mental health problem.
- Once again a tight safety net should be applied and you really have to be sure there is no overt suicidal or self-harm intent and there is an adequate support structure in place at home.
- Short-term medication options include:
  - propranolol (40mg every 8 hours) for anxiety and panic attacks
  - diazepam (2mg every 8 hours) for anxiety and agitation
  - lorazepam (0.5–2.0mg every 8 hours) for anxiety and agitation
  - promethazine 25mg at night for insomnia and agitation
  - zopiclone 3.75mg at night for insomnia
  - amitriptyline 10mg at night for insomnia.
- Avoid starting long-term medication such as SSRIs, as they can exacerbate symptoms in the first few weeks and patients will require monitoring, which is not usually possible in an OOH or urgent care setting.
- Consider emailing a letter to the patient's regular GP highlighting your concerns and requesting a follow-up.
- Local improving access to psychological therapies (IAPT) services may also be available and patients can self-refer.

Risk factors and red flag features in patients presenting with suicidal ideation

- A previous history of self-harm or attempted suicide
- A history of mental illness such as a personality disorder or psychosis
- Disengagement from mental health services
- A family member or friend who has died by suicide
- Male (often men may not disclose suicidal intent)
- Suicidal thoughts with preparation or a plan put in place
- A perception of lack of support
- A high degree of negative thoughts or helplessness
- Life stresses such as bereavement or financial difficulties
- Alcohol or drug abuse

- Patients who have suicidal or self-harm intent require referral to ED or the on-call community psychiatric nurse (CPN), crisis team or the community mental health team (CMHT).

Delirium (sudden confusion)

Presentation[2],[3]

- In the elderly this is commonly due to an infection such as a UTI.
- Other causes include any acute medical or surgical problem, drug and alcohol intoxication or withdrawal.
- Hypercalcaemia is also a cause of acute confusion and should be suspected in all patients with malignant neoplastic disease, especially if there is metastatic spread to bone.
- It is essential to assess, identify and treat the underlying cause of delirium.
- Acute on chronic confusion can also occur, and again it is important to identify a trigger.
- Try to obtain a history from relatives or friends and determine what the baseline is for the patient.

Patients with mild symptoms who are systemically well and where the aetiology is known can be managed over the phone and medication prescribed remotely.

In cases where the history or diagnosis is unclear a face-to-face assessment should be arranged.

Assessment

- A full examination including a urinalysis should be undertaken.
- A mini mental status examination can help quantify cognitive impairment.

Management[3],[4]

- If an obvious cause cannot be identified then the patient should be referred to the on-call medical team.
- Haloperidol 0.5–1.0mg or lorazepam 0.5mg can be used to treat anxiety and agitation in the interim.

Common causes of delirium

- Infections
- Acute medical conditions, e.g. stroke
- Acute surgical conditions, e.g. peritonitis
- Drug or alcohol intoxication or withdrawal
- Metabolic or endocrine imbalances
- Brain injury

Acute psychosis

Presentation

- Acute psychotic episodes present with hallucinations, delusions and a loss of reality.
- The patient may already have a history of psychosis and early warning signs of a relapse include social withdrawal, paranoid ideas, suspiciousness, a drop in personal hygiene, loss of job, changes in mood and sleep disturbances.

Management

- This requires admission to hospital and a formal mental health assessment.
- Patients with acute psychosis require specialist input and should be referred directly to the on-call psychiatry team or community mental health team.
- The ED is considered a place of safety and patients should be assessed there by an appropriate multidisciplinary team.
- Medication to control symptoms can be prescribed in the short term and includes lorazepam 0.5–1.0mg PO for anxiety every 8 hours or haloperidol 0.75–1.5mg PO every 8 hours[5].

Mental capacity

Presentation

- The first principle of the Mental Capacity Act 2005[6] is that a person is assumed to have capacity unless proven otherwise. It applies to people aged 16 years and over.
- For people younger than 16 years capacity should be assessed on an individual basis.
- Ideally mental capacity should be assessed face-to-face.
- In an OOH setting it is not uncommon for paramedics to call to seek advice regarding patients who have refused to go to hospital. Often the paramedics will have assessed capacity and will require advice and guidance on whether the patient can be managed at home.
- Bear in mind that capacity can fluctuate and is also decision-specific, i.e. a person may have capacity to make a decision about one aspect of their life but not another.
- Therefore, when assessing a person's capacity it is important to assess the person in 'real time' and in the context of the situation.
- A person may lack capacity due to physical illness, brain injury, learning difficulties, dementia, mental health illness or due to alcohol or drug intoxication or withdrawal.

Assessment[7]

- First consider if the patient has an impairment which may affect capacity. If not, the patient is assumed to have capacity and the decision made by the patient should be accepted even if it is considered unwise.
- If the patient does have an impairment which may affect capacity, consider if this impairment is temporary and whether waiting until the person is better will allow the person to make a decision.

- Consider any adjuncts such as information leaflets or sign language which may assist the patient in making a decision.
- If the impairment is considered permanent and all measures to assist the patient in making a decision have been exhausted, then assess the patient's capacity, taking into account the following:
  - is the patient able to understand the information provided?
  - is the patient able to retain the information long enough to make a decision?
  - is the patient able to consider the pros and cons of any decision they make?
  - is the patient able to communicate this decision?
- If the answer to all of the above questions is yes, then the patient has capacity.
- If the answer to any one of the above questions is no, the patient does not have capacity and all decisions should be made in the patient's best interests.

Management[8]

- If a patient lacks mental capacity and is unlikely to regain this, then all decisions should be made in the best interests of the patient.
- Enquire about any advance directives or plans; these may be with the patient or the patient's regular GP.
- Speak to the patient's next of kin, carers and – if the patient has one – their attorney or court-appointed deputy, to ascertain what the patient's wishes were before loss of capacity.
- Encourage the patient to participate in the decision-making process and try to establish what the patient's wishes are.
- Consider the least restrictive option, i.e. the option that will result in the least loss of the patient's liberties and freedom.
- If necessary seek legal advice from the clinical lead at your employing organisation or your indemnity provider.

Summary for mental health

- Avoid prescribing long-term or large supplies of medication to patients who present with acute mental health problems.
- Consider emailing a letter to the patient's regular GP.
- Infections are a common cause of confusion in the elderly.

References

1. NICE (updated 2020) *Generalised anxiety disorder and panic disorder in adults: management* [CG113]. Available at: www.nice.org.uk/guidance/cg113

2. NICE (updated 2023) *Delirium: prevention, diagnosis and management* [CG103]. Available at: www.nice.org.uk/guidance/cg103

3. Kalish, V.B., Gillham, J.E. and Unwin, B.K. (2014) Delirium in older persons: evaluation and management. *Am Fam Physician*, **90(3):** 150–8.

4. NICE (revised 2023) *Delirium*. Scenario: Management. Available at: https://cks.nice.org.uk/delirium#!scenario

5. BNF (no date) *Psychoses and related disorders*. Advice of Royal College of Psychiatrists of antipsychotic drugs above BNF upper limit. Available at: https://bnf.nice.org.uk/treatment-summary/psychoses-and-related-disorders.html

6. Office of the Public Guardian (updated 2020) *Mental Capacity Act Code of Practice*. Available at: www.gov.uk/government/publications/mental-capacity-act-code-of-practice

7. BMA (updated 2024) *Mental Capacity Act Toolkit*. Available at: www.bma.org.uk/advice-and-support/ethics/adults-who-lack-capacity/mental-capacity-act-toolkit

8. NHS (no date) Mental Capacity Act. Available at: www.nhs.uk/conditions/social-care-and-support-guide/making-decisions-for-someone-else/mental-capacity-act/

16

Chapter 16: **Poisoning, overdose and foreign body ingestion**

"All things are poisons, for there is nothing without poisonous qualities. It is only the dose which makes a thing poison."
Paracelsus

Assessment of patients with poisoning, overdose and foreign body ingestion

Telephone

- A detailed history should always be taken over the phone.
- Determine what substance has been taken.
- Enquire whether this was deliberate or accidental.
- Enquire about time of ingestion or exposure and the duration of exposure.
- Ask about any evidence to confirm the quantity of substance ingested, e.g. empty pill packets or empty bottles.
- If the patient is a child, speak to the parent or guardian.
- Enquire about past medical problems, including any mental health problems.
- The carer or patient may be able to check basic observations.

Once a detailed history has been taken it will often become apparent if the patient requires a referral to ED (for investigations or monitoring) or can be managed at home.

If there is any doubt, a face-to-face assessment should be arranged.

Poisoning

Presentation

- The initial call may be from the patient or a parent or next of kin.
- If possible, speak to the patient.
- Take a detailed history over the phone.
- People who call suspecting their drinks have been spiked (i.e. alcohol or drugs have been added to someone's drink without their knowledge) should be advised to contact the police as soon as possible, because spiking someone's drink is a criminal offence.

Assessment

- Enquire about any current symptoms, especially breathing problems, chest pain, palpitations, vomiting, seizures and altered consciousness, as these should be considered red flag features[1].

- If assessing the patient face-to-face, a full set of observations should be taken.
- The triaging clinician can access TOXBASE[2]; this is an online database which can provide information to healthcare professionals who are managing patients who have ingested or been exposed to toxic substances. Access to TOXBASE will usually be provided by the hospital Trust or the OOH employing organisation.
- The National Poisons Information service (NPIS)[3] can be contacted to discuss complex cases regarding ingestion of multiple toxins. The service is available 24 hours a day via the central UK number 0344 892 0111.
- A face-to-face assessment is rarely required in primary care as in the majority of cases patients will fall into two groups: those requiring an immediate admission to hospital, and those who can be managed at home with telephone advice, e.g. they have taken an extra dose of their medication.
- If the decision is to provide telephone advice then it is essential patients are provided with appropriate safety-netting advice. This should include advice on what symptoms to look out for, and that if there are any concerns whatsoever the patient should call 111 or seek medical attention.
- Determine and assess any safeguarding concerns.

Management

- If the patient is having symptoms they should be referred to hospital; if there are red flag features then an emergency ambulance should be arranged.
- Those who have taken deliberate overdose should be referred to ED. If the patient refuses, an assessment of their mental capacity should be made and if necessary, an admission under the Mental Health Act can be undertaken.
- Certain substances, such as salicylates, paracetamol and tricyclic antidepressants, may present with delayed onset of symptoms; these patients should be referred to hospital if large amounts have been ingested.

Foreign body ingestion

Presentation

- This is most common in children aged 6 months to 6 years[4], with coins being the most common object ingested.
- 80% of ingested foreign bodies will pass through the GI tract[5].
- Presentation is variable and will very much depend on if and where the object is lodged.
- Foreign bodies lodged at the oropharyngeal junction will present with discomfort, pain, dysphagia, odynophagia, drooling and potentially dyspnoea.
- Foreign bodies lodged at the gastro-oesophageal junction will present with pain, vomiting, abdominal bloating and potentially features of GI bleeding such as melaena.
- Features of GI perforation include severe chest or abdominal pain, bloating, dyspnoea, melaena, haematemesis, tachycardia, hypotension and collapse.
- GI perforation is likely if the foreign body has sharp edges or a sharp point, such as a toothpick.

- Patients who have swallowed a foreign body will require an ED assessment; if there are severe symptoms consider an emergency ambulance transfer.

Assessment

- If you are seeing the patient face-to-face, ensure observations are assessed and recorded.
- Assess for any complications such as GI perforation.
- Radio-opaque foreign bodies, e.g. coins and steak bones, can be visualised on X-rays.
- CT imaging can also locate foreign bodies and identify complications.

Management

- Foreign bodies in the oropharynx which are visible may be removed carefully using forceps.
- Any foreign bodies that are lodged below the oropharynx will require removal via endoscopy, and a referral to hospital is warranted.
- If there are signs of complications such as GI perforation, or if the patient is systemically unwell, transfer to hospital should be via emergency ambulance.
- Consider safeguarding issues, especially if there are repeated presentations of ingested foreign bodies.

Summary for poisoning, overdose and foreign body ingestion

- Often it will be apparent over the phone if the patient requires a direct referral to ED.
- Utilise appropriate online resources such as TOXBASE.
- Consider safeguarding issues.

References

1. NICE (revised 2024) *Poisoning or overdose*. CKS. Available at: https://cks.nice.org.uk/topics/poisoning-or-overdose/

2. TOXBASE: www.toxbase.org/

3. National Poisons Information Service: www.npis.org/index.html

4. Ambe, P., Weber, S.A., Schauer, M. and Knoefel, W.T. (2012) Swallowed foreign bodies in adults. *Dtsch Arztebl Int*, **109(50):** 869–875.

5. Willacy, H. (updated 2021) *Swallowed foreign bodies: causes, symptoms and treatment*. Available at: https://patient.info/doctor/swallowed-foreign-bodies#ref-2

17

Chapter 17: **Dermatology**

"A thick skin is a gift from God."
Konrad Adenauer

Assessment of patients presenting with acute skin conditions

Telephone

- A detailed history can be taken over the phone; however, it can be difficult to diagnose skin conditions by history alone.
- Enquire about blanching and non-blanching rashes.
- Enquire about associated symptoms such as pyrexia or pruritus.
- Patients who have a pyrexia, are unwell and have a non-blanching rash should be referred to hospital via ambulance, as these features suggest meningococcal sepsis.
- Enquire about previous episodes and how they were managed.
- Dermnet NZ (www.dermnetnz.org) is an excellent online resource providing free access to images of almost all skin conditions.

Video consultation may assist, but often this will depend on the quality of the camera, computer screen and internet connection. Photographs will be of more use and the patient may be able to email these or send via software programs such as AccuRx.

Face-to-face

Face-to-face assessment would be required in the following situations:

- The diagnosis is not obvious from telephone triage and images.
- There are associated symptoms causing distress.
- The patient has systemic symptoms such as pyrexia.

Have a low threshold for assessing children face-to-face.

Cellulitis

Presentation

- This is an infection of the skin and underlying tissues.
- It is usually caused by a break in the skin which allows the bacterium *Staphylococcus aureus* to penetrate.
- The affected area will look red and be painful.
- Enquire about systemic symptoms such as pyrexia, malaise, nausea and vomiting.

Patients who have mild and recurrent episodes of cellulitis can be prescribed antibiotics over the phone. If the diagnosis is in doubt, a video consultation may help.

For patients who are unwell or where the diagnosis is unclear, a face-to-face consultation should be conducted.

Assessment

- The affected area will be painful, erythematous, blistering, shiny, warm and tender (*Fig. 17.1*).
- Check general observations and markers for sepsis which would indicate systemic infection.

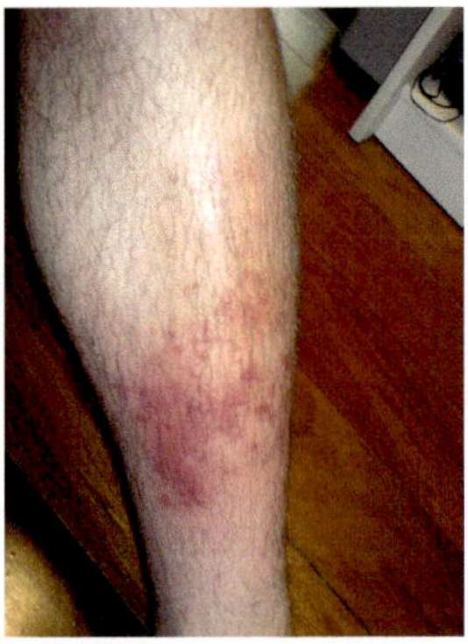

Fig. 17.1: Cellulitis of the left leg.

Reproduced from https://en.wikipedia.org/wiki/Cellulitis under a CC BY-SA 3.0 licence (photo by Rafael Lopez).

Management

- Treatment is with oral antibiotics, with the first line being flucloxacillin 250–500mg QDS × 5–7 days.
- Co-amoxiclav 625mg PO TDS × 5–7 days should be given to patients who have cellulitis around the eyes and nose.
- Erythromycin 250–500mg QDS × 5–7 days or clarithromycin 250–500mg QDS × 5–7 days can be prescribed to those with a penicillin allergy.
- Occasionally more than 7 days of treatment may be required.
- The erythema associated with cellulitis can take several weeks to resolve.
- For patients who are systemically unwell, immunocompromised, unable to take oral antibiotics or showing no response to oral antibiotics, admission to hospital should be arranged.

Eczema (dermatitis)

The two terms eczema and dermatitis are interchangeable and refer to inflammation of the skin.

Presentation

- There are several types of dermatitis including atopic (*Fig. 17.2*), contact and irritant dermatitis.
- Patches of the skin will appear inflamed and will be pruritic.

Patients may have had previous episodes and therefore may only require a prescription for topical corticosteroids, which can be issued remotely.

Management

- Treatment is based on emollients and topical corticosteroids such as hydrocortisone (mild), clobetasone (moderate) and mometasone (potent).
- It is important to specify the duration of treatment on the prescription.

- Creams are water-based and ointments are oil-based. Ointments will stay on the skin longer and will trap moisture, so are preferable in those with dry skin.
- Pastes will form a protective barrier, and can also be infused into bandages.
- Signs of infection (purulent discharge or exudate) should be observed for, and if absent this should be documented.
- If patches appear to be infected then oral antibiotics should be prescribed.
- If the patient is systemically unwell (tachycardia, pyrexia), as can be the case with erythroderma and exfoliative dermatitis, the patient should be referred to the on-call medical team.

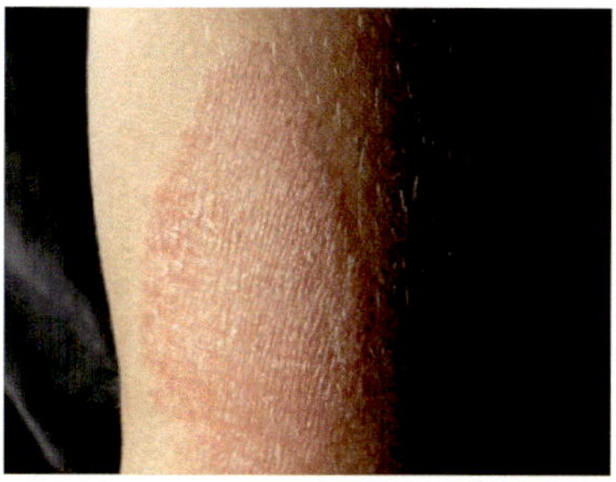

Fig. 17.2: Atopic dermatitis.

Reproduced from https://commons.wikimedia.org/wiki/File:Dermatite_o_eczema_atopico_avambraccio_2015.jpg under a CC BY-SA 3.0 licence (photo by G.steph.rocket).

Topical corticosteroid potency:

- Hydrocortisone 1% (mild)
- Clobetasone 0.05% (moderate)
- Betamethasone 0.1% (potent)
- Mometasone 0.1% (very potent)
- Triamcinolone 0.1% (very potent)

Erysipelas

Presentation

- This is a form of cellulitis affecting the upper dermis; however, it is much more serious.
- It is caused by *Streptococcus pyogenes* and is more common in infants, the elderly and the immunocompromised.
- Erysipelas can affect any part of the skin but is more common on the face (*Fig. 17.3*) and legs.
- Patients can be systemically very unwell, exhibiting markers of sepsis.

As patients can be very unwell and the condition can be difficult to differentiate from severe cellulitis, a face-to-face assessment is recommended.

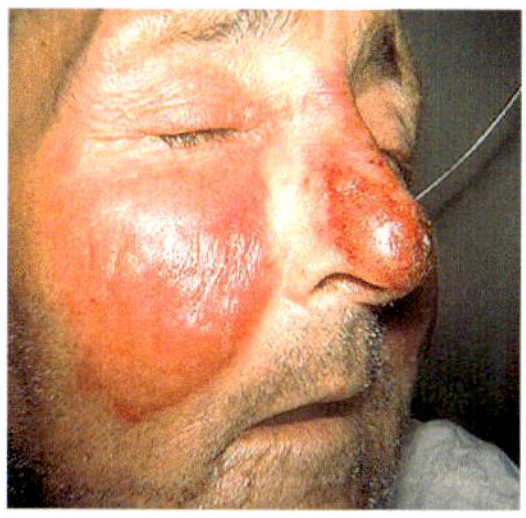

Fig. 17.3: Erysipelas affecting the face; note the well-demarcated border and elevation.

Reproduced from https://en.wikipedia.org/wiki/Erysipelas Public domain (photo by CDC).

Assessment

- Skin lesions are erythematous, raised, well-demarcated, painful and very tender.

- Vesicles, bullae, petechiae and necrosis may also feature.
- The well-defined margins and elevation assist in differentiating erysipelas from cellulitis.

Management

- Patients with mild features, who are systemically well and do not exhibit any skin necrosis, can be managed with oral antibiotics.
- The drug of choice is phenoxymethylpenicillin 500mg QDS × 10 days[1]. For those who have a penicillin allergy a macrolide such as clarithromycin 500mg BD × 10 days can be prescribed.
- Patients who are systemically unwell or have features of skin necrosis should be referred urgently to the on-call medical team.

Erythema migrans and Lyme disease

Presentation

- This is an erythematous rash, often described as having a 'bull's eye' appearance.
- It is a circular lesion, with a red ring, central clearing and a 'bull's eye' in the middle (*Fig. 17.4*).
- It is an expanding lesion and will increase in diameter over the course of a few days.
- It is asymptomatic.
- Erythema migrans usually appears within 4 weeks of a tick bite, but can appear up to 3 months later.
- The rash itself is completely harmless but it can be a manifestation of Lyme disease, an infectious disease caused by the bacteria *Borrelia burgdorferi* which is transmitted via ticks.

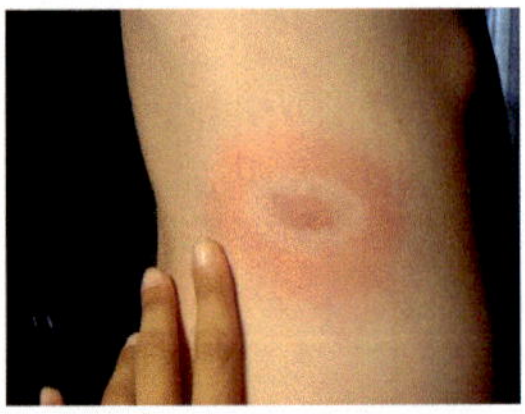

Fig. 17.4: Erythema migrans rash – although asymptomatic, it can be a feature of Lyme disease.

Photographs or a video consultation will usually be enough to confirm the diagnosis of erythema migrans. Patients who have erythema migrans and no other symptoms may benefit from serology. Early treatment of Lyme disease is recommended to prevent long-term sequelae.

If there are systemic symptoms then a face-to-face assessment should be arranged.

Assessment

- Erythema migrans is asymptomatic; however, patients with Lyme disease may have pyrexia, malaise, fatigue, lymphadenopathy, aching joints, myalgia and headaches.
- Organ-specific sequelae can occur, including nerve palsies, neuropsychiatric problems, neuropathy, meningitis, pericarditis, heart block, uveitis and keratitis.

Management[2]

- All under 18-year-olds with suspected Lyme disease should be discussed with a specialist.
- There is an argument that children with erythema migrans and no other symptoms do not require treatment; however, in clinical practice specialist advice from the on-call paediatricians should be sought.
- In adults with erythema migrans and no other symptoms serology should be considered. If serological testing is unavailable then the recommendation is to treat based on the clinical picture.
- Patients with Lyme disease and organ-specific features should be started on antibiotics. Options are doxycycline 100mg PO BD or 200mg PO OD × 21 days, or amoxicillin 1g PO TDS × 21 days.
- Patients with organ-specific or focal symptoms should be discussed with a specialist to determine the need for IV antibiotics.

Folliculitis

Presentation

- Folliculitis refers to inflammation of the hair follicles (*Fig. 17.5*).
- It can occur due to trauma but is commonly associated with a *Staphylococcus aureus* infection.

Very rarely will a face-to-face consultation be required, as the diagnosis can usually be made from photographs or a video consultation.

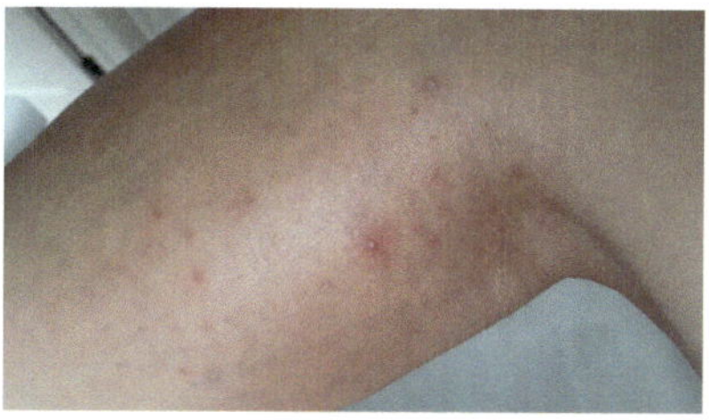

Fig. 17.5: Folliculitis of the leg.

Assessment

- Erythematous papules and pustules are seen over the affected areas.
- Patients will be systemically well.

Management

- Treatment is with oral antibiotics such as flucloxacillin 250–500mg QDS × 5–7 days or clarithromycin 250–500mg BD × 5–7 days.
- A topical corticosteroid cream will assist in alleviating inflammation.

Guttate psoriasis

Presentation

- Guttate psoriasis is a form of psoriasis that develops after a streptococcal throat infection.

- Other triggers include injury to the skin, stress and certain drugs such as anti-malaria medication. Onset is usually a few days to weeks after the original trigger.

It can be difficult to diagnose over the phone so a video or face-to-face consultation may be needed to establish the diagnosis.

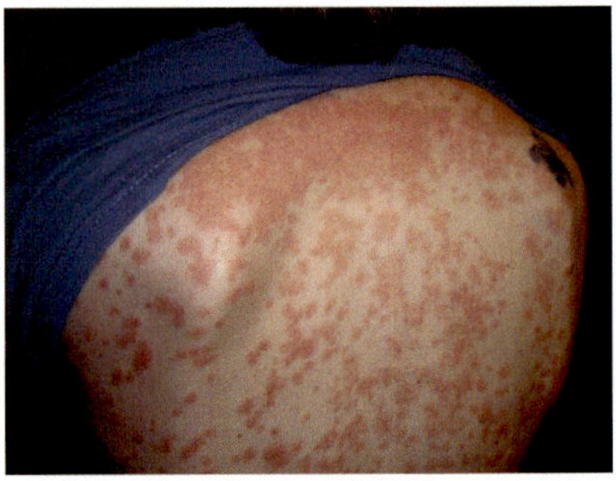

Fig. 17.6: Guttate psoriasis.

Reproduced from https://en.wikipedia.org/wiki/Guttate_psoriasis under a CC BY-SA 4.0 licence (photo by Bobjgalindo).

Assessment

- Red scaly teardrop or discoid-type lesions develop all over the skin. They have a characteristic scaly appearance (*Fig. 17.6*).
- It may resemble pityriasis rosea; however, the lesions tend to be thicker and there is no herald patch.
- Although the eruption may be alarming, patients will be well.

Management

- Acute eruptions can be managed with emollients and topical corticosteroids.

Hand, foot and mouth disease

Presentation [3]

- This usually occurs in children and is caused by the Coxsackie virus.
- As the name suggests, the rash affects the hand and feet, with lesions in or around the mouth as well (*Fig. 17.7*).

As most people affected by this are well, a telephone consultation or video consultation is usually enough to provide reassurance.

Assessment

- Erythematous blanching papules are characteristically found on the hands, feet, around the mouth and nappy area.
- Lesions can also be seen inside the mouth.
- It may be accompanied by a high temperature and coryzal symptoms.
- The rash and infection is self-limiting, usually lasting 10 days.

Management [4]

- This centres around symptom control with the use of analgesia, antipyretics, mouth gels and oral hydration.

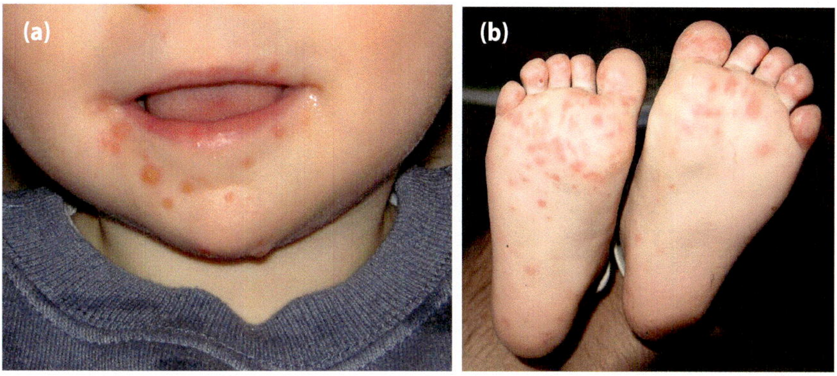

Fig. 17.7: Hand, foot and mouth disease lesions (a) around the mouth; (b) on the feet.

(a) reproduced from https://commons.wikimedia.org/wiki/File:Hand_Foot_Mouth_Disease.png (photo by Midgley DJ); (b) reproduced from https://commons.wikimedia.org/wiki/File:Hand_foot_and_mouth_disease_on_child_feet (photo by Ngufra);

Herpes simplex virus

Presentation

- Although lesions can occur anywhere on the body, a general rule is that oral lesions (*Fig. 17.8*) tend to be caused by HSV I and genital lesions tend to be caused by HSV II.
- The virus is spread by direct contact.
- It may remain dormant for an unknown period of time, with active infections triggered off by the onset of an acute illness or spontaneously.
- Early warning signs include tingling, itching and a burning sensation.
- The rash will usually resemble a crop of vesicles and be present for 7–10 days.

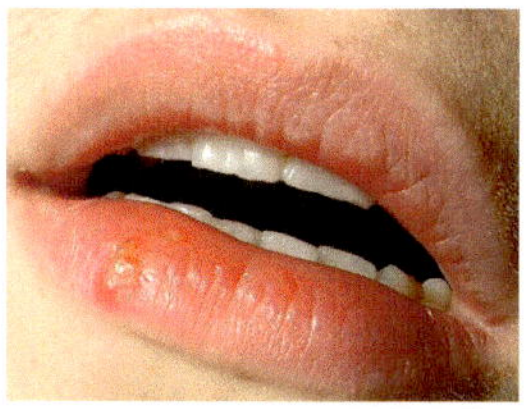

Fig. 17.8: Herpes simplex I infection (herpes labialis).

Reproduced from https://commons.wikimedia.org/wiki/File:Herpes_labialis.jpg Public domain (photo by Metju12).

Patients will usually present with recurrent episodes so will be aware of the cause; in such cases patients can be referred to their local pharmacist for topical medication.

Management

- The treatment is topical aciclovir (available over the counter from a pharmacy) or oral aciclovir, given 200mg five times a day × 7 days.
- It is important to look for features of superimposed bacterial infection, as this will require oral antibiotics.
- Genital herpes in pregnant women close to the time of delivery is an indication for caesarean section.

Herpes zoster (shingles)

Presentation

- This occurs due to reactivation of the varicella zoster virus which can remain dormant within the body for several years.
- It is more common in the elderly and immunocompromised.
- Pain or a tingling sensation may typically precede the rash, which presents as erythematous vesicles (blisters) in a dermatomal distribution (*Fig. 17.9*).
- Importantly, the rash will not cross the midline.

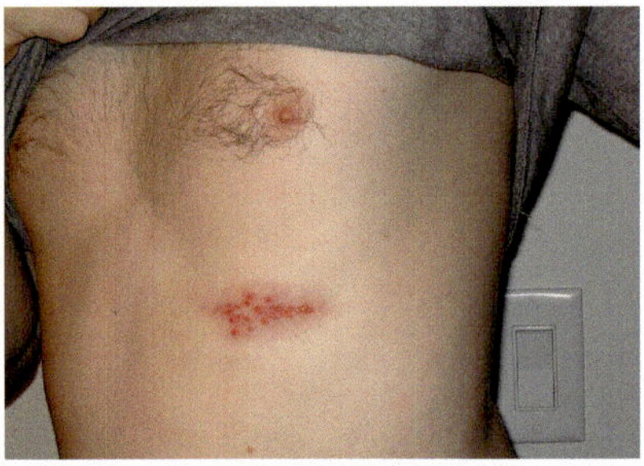

Fig. 17.9: A shingles (herpes zoster) outbreak on the chest.

Reproduced from https://commons.wikimedia.org/wiki/File:Shingles_on_the_chest.jpg under a CC BY 3.0 licence (photo by Preston Hunt).

Management[5]

- Oral antiviral administration within the first 72 hours of the rash has been shown to reduce the duration of symptoms and the likelihood of developing complications.
- Aciclovir 800mg PO five times a day × 7 days is the drug of choice.
- Ideally the rash should be kept covered to reduce the risk of spread.
- Pain can be managed with the use of paracetamol, ibuprofen, codeine and amitriptyline.

Impetigo

Presentation[6]

- This is a localised skin infection caused by *Staphylococcus aureus*.
- It commonly presents in children.
- The two types are bullous (with large blisters) or non-bullous (red and crusting; *Fig 17.10*).
- It is a highly contagious but benign and often self-limiting condition.

Some patients and parents will be familiar with the condition and there may be a history of previous episodes. In such cases and provided the patient is well, a prescription can usually be issued over the phone. However, if there is any doubt then photographs may help to establish the diagnosis.

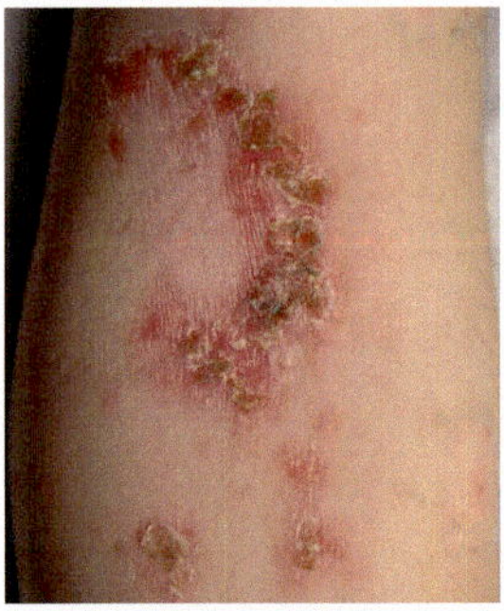

Fig. 17.10: Non-bullous impetigo of the elbow.

Reproduced from https://commons.wikimedia.org/wiki/File:Impetigo_elbow.jpg under a CC BY-SA 3.0 licence (photo by Evanherk).

Management[6],[7]

- Although topical fusidic acid cream can be applied, there is little evidence to suggest it makes a difference when treating mild cases.
- Widespread impetigo should be treated with oral antibiotics such as flucloxacillin 250–500mg PO QDS or clarithromycin 250–500mg PO BD × 5–7 days.

Measles

Presentation[8]

- This usually occurs in children but can present in adults who are not immunised.
- Presenting features include a high temperature, coryzal symptoms and sore eyes.

People with measles can be acutely unwell and often the rash can be difficult to diagnose over the phone or via video consultation. As a result a face-to-face assessment may be required.

Assessment

- Check general observations.
- Assess for complications such as pneumonia or encephalitis.
- The rash, which has a purplish hue, usually starts behind the ears or on the face and spreads down the body (*Fig. 17.11*).
- The presence of Koplik spots (white pinprick spots; *Fig. 17.12*) on the buccal mucosa is pathognomonic.

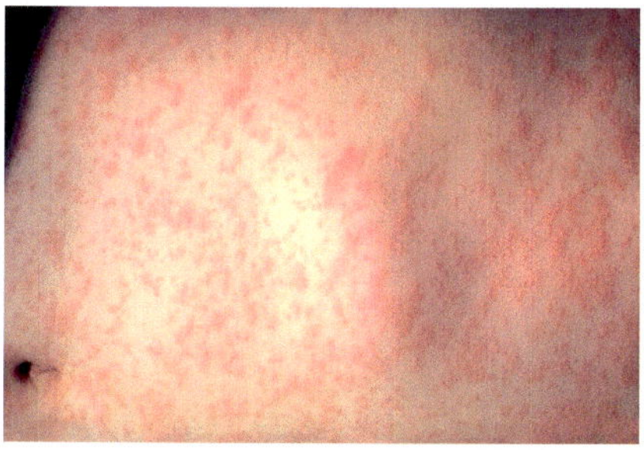

Fig. 17.11: Maculopapular rash of measles on the torso.

Reproduced from Centers for Disease Control and Prevention's Public Health Image Library (PHIL). Public domain (photo by Heinz F. Eichenwald).

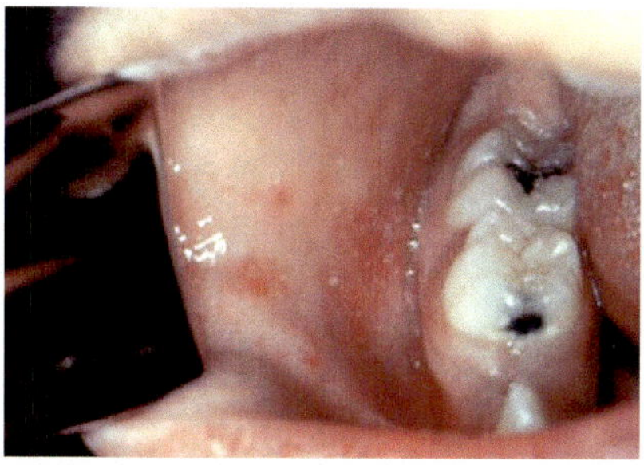

Fig. 17.12: Koplik spots on the buccal mucosa.

Reproduced from Centers for Disease Control and Prevention's Public Health Image Library (PHIL). Public domain.

Management

- There is no treatment for measles; the infection itself is self-limiting, often lasting 10 days. Management is supportive with the use of analgesia, antipyretics and oral hydration.

- Patients presenting with complications should be referred to the nearest ED.
- Confirmation of measles is done via buccal scrapings and serology.

Note on measles

In the UK measles is a notifiable disease and any suspected cases should be referred to the local health protection team.

Meningococcal septicaemia

Presentation[9]

- This is a separate entity to meningitis; patients will not have a headache, neck stiffness and photophobia.
- Those affected will become very unwell, very quickly.

Any patient who has a non-blanching rash and is acutely unwell should have an emergency ambulance arranged for immediate transfer to hospital.

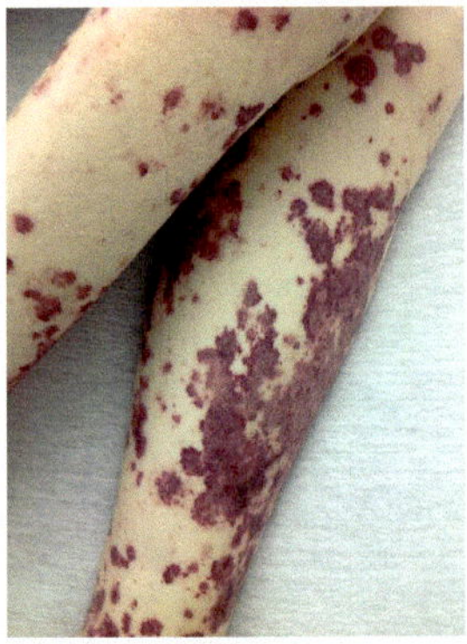

Fig. 17.13: Petechial rash associated with meningococcal septicaemia.

Reproduced from https://commons.wikimedia.org/wiki/File:Petechial_rash.JPG under a CC BY-SA 3.0 licence (photo by DrFO.jr.Tn).

Assessment

- There will be features of sepsis, including a high or low temperature, drowsiness, lethargy and poor feeding.
- The patient will be systemically unwell, with tachycardia and hypotension indicating hypovolaemic shock.
- The rash associated with meningococcal septicaemia is petechial (*Fig. 17.13*) or purpuric, i.e. non-blanching in nature.
- It characteristically starts distally and works its way up the body, hence it is essential to assess the whole skin and not just central areas.
- Patients may also have conjunctival petechiae.

Management

All patients with suspected meningococcal septicaemia should be given benzyl penicillin IM if available (300mg for patients <1 year old, 600mg for those aged 1–9 years, and 1200mg for those over 10 years) and transferred to hospital immediately.

Features of meningococcal septicaemia

- Can result in sudden deterioration and can kill within hours
- Petechial (non-blanching) rash
- Rash starts peripherally
- Conjunctival petechiae
- Lethargy
- Drowsiness
- Poor feeding
- A very high or low temperature
- Tachycardia
- Hypotension

Non-specific viral rash

Presentation

- It is difficult to identify the exact aetiology of a viral rash, hence the term 'non-specific viral rash' or exanthem.
- The usual suspects are respiratory syncytial virus, parvovirus, adenovirus, rotavirus and Epstein–Barr virus.
- There may or may not be an associated pyrexia, coryzal symptoms and GI symptoms.

If the patient is well and the clinician confident the rash is blanching and benign, then telephone advice will usually suffice. However, if there are any doubts then a video consultation or a face-to-face consultation is recommended.

Assessment

- The rash will usually start on the torso and spread outwards.
- Characteristically it will be macular, erythematous and blanching; affecting the torso, arms, legs and face.
- General observations will usually be within normal range.

Rash: blanching vs. non-blanching

One of the most important defining features of a rash is whether it is blanching or non-blanching. The presence or absence of this feature must be documented in the patient's medical records at the time of assessment. Non-blanching rashes require further investigations.

Management

- The rash is benign and self-limiting.
- It can take 2 weeks to clear.
- Patients should be reassured and advised about sinister features to look out for such as a non-blanching rash, and to return if they have any concerns.

Parvovirus B19 infection (slapped cheek syndrome, fifth disease)

Presentation

- This will usually affect young children between the ages of 5 and 12 years.
- Seasonal outbreaks from winter to spring may occur.
- A bright red rash appears on the cheeks (hence the name slapped cheek syndrome); this may be associated with a high temperature and a blanching, erythematous and pruritic rash on the body similar to a non-specific viral rash (*Fig. 17.14*).

Most patients can be managed over the phone with advice; however, if there are systemic symptoms and the diagnosis is unclear, a face-to-face assessment should be considered.

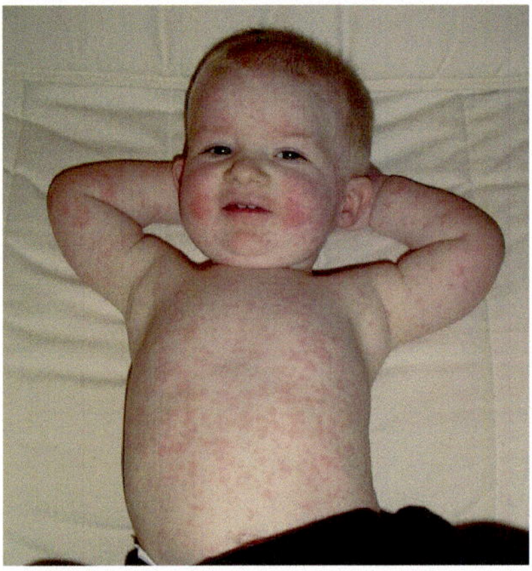

Fig. 17.14: The rash associated with parvovirus B19 infection – note the concentration on the cheeks.

Reproduced from https://commons.wikimedia.org/w/index.php?curid=1857945 Public domain (photo by Andrew Kerr).

Management

- This is a benign, self-limiting condition, with the rash lasting for 10–14 days.
- Management is supportive, with paracetamol, fluids and reassurance.
- Moisturising creams and antihistamines will help with pruritus.
- Those with parvovirus infection should be advised to avoid contact with pregnant women (see below).
- Rare complications include aplastic anaemia, arthropathy and neuropathy.

Parvovirus B19 infection in pregnant women [10]

- Although most women are asymptomatic, 3% of women can suffer complications such as miscarriage, foetal anaemia and foetal demise.
- The risk of complications is higher in the first trimester. After 20 weeks of gestation the risk disappears.
- Specialist advice should be sought when managing pregnant women with a suspected parvovirus infection – serology testing and regular ultrasound examinations may be required.

Pityriasis rosea

Presentation [11]

- This is a relatively common but underdiagnosed benign skin condition.
- It mainly affects young adults.

- The exact aetiology is unknown; however, it is believed to be due to a viral infection.
- Some people may be unwell with coryzal symptoms a few days prior to the onset of skin manifestations.
- The rash is characterised by a 'herald patch' which appears a few days before the more widespread rash manifests.

Although patients will be well, it can be difficult to diagnose the rash over the phone, primarily because patients may struggle to identify the herald patch and also because the rash has a similar appearance to certain types of psoriasis. In such cases a video or face-to-face consultation may be required.

Assessment

- The herald patch is a discoid red scaly lesion a few centimetres in diameter.
- Patients usually present when the widespread rash has appeared (*Fig. 17.15*).
- The rash consists of 2–10cm-diameter red scaly lesions, mainly on the torso but also affecting the limbs and groin areas.
- The rash can be pruritic.
- General observations will be normal and the patient will be well.

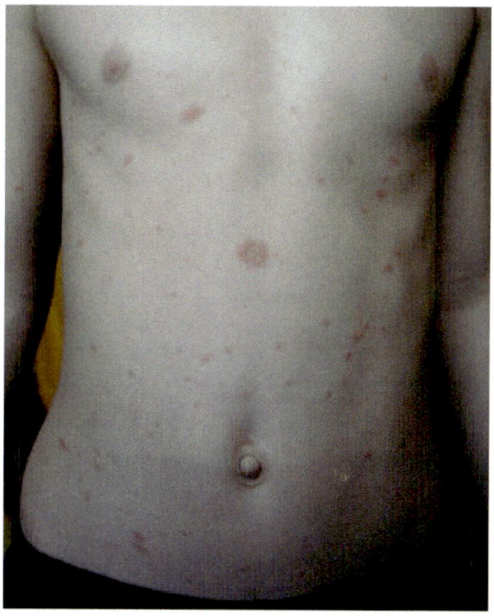

Fig. 17.15: Pityriasis rosea rash – notice the herald patch in the centre.

Management

- Options to control symptoms are emollients, oral antihistamines and topical corticosteroid creams.
- It can take up to 16 weeks to resolve, and patients should be reassured that it is considered non-contagious.
- Pityriasis rosea in the first 15 weeks of pregnancy has been associated with complications such as miscarriage and premature delivery, and therefore advice from an obstetrician should be sought.

Pityriasis (tinea) versicolor

Presentation

- As these lesions tend to be asymptomatic, patients will rarely present acutely.
- Often they are more noticeable after prolonged sun exposure, hence presentations tend to be more common after summer or a holiday in the sun.

Patients will be well and face-to-face consultation is not required; the diagnosis can be made on video consultation or using photographs.

Assessment

- The patient will be well.
- The skin on the torso will be covered in hypo- (*Fig. 17.16*) or hyperpigmented macules.

Management

- The treatment is topical ketoconazole or selenium sulphide shampoo. Ketoconazole cream can also be used. If topical antifungal treatment fails then oral fluconazole 50mg once daily for 2 weeks can be prescribed.

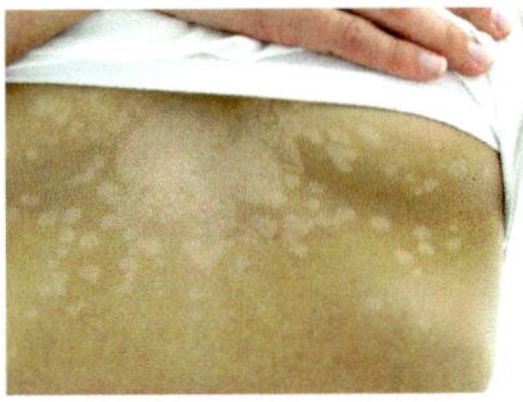

Fig. 17.16: Tinea versicolor.

Reproduced from https://commons.wikimedia.org/wiki/File:Tinea_versicolor1.jpg under a CC-BY-SA-2.0 licence (photo by Sarahrosenau).

Tinea (dermatophyte, ringworm)

Presentation

- This presents with an intensely pruritic lesion, discoid in shape with an erythematous raised border and central clearing (*Fig. 17.17*).
- It can occur anywhere on the body and is named according to the area affected: corporis (body), cruris (groin) and pedis (feet).
- Patients will be generally well.

Patients will be well and face-to-face consultation is not required – the diagnosis can be made on video consultation or using photographs.

Management

- The treatment is topical clotrimazole 1% or miconazole 2% cream applied twice a day × 4 weeks.
- If the lesions fail to respond then oral fluconazole 50mg once daily × 2 weeks can be prescribed.
- Differentials include discoid eczema where there will be multiple lesions with a relapsing–remitting history of inflammation of the skin, and granuloma annulare which tends to be non-pruritic and has an insidious onset.
- Widespread granuloma annulare may be associated with underlying conditions such as diabetes mellitus, and patients who present with widespread lesions should be investigated for this.

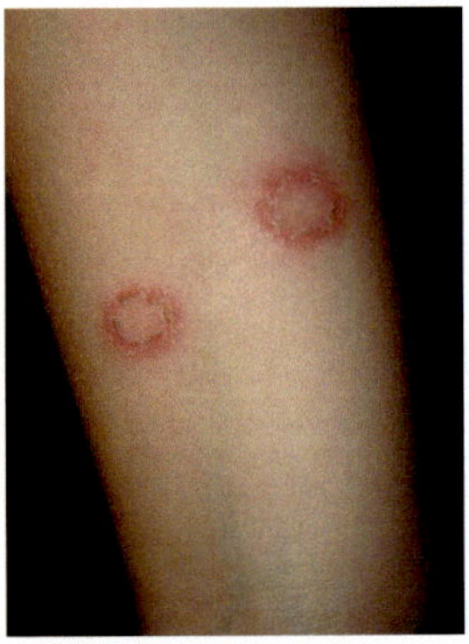

Fig. 17.17: Ringworm infection of the arm.

Reproduced from https://commons.wikimedia.org/wiki/File:Herpes_circin%C3%A9_01.jpg under a CC BY-SA 3.0 licence (photo by Grook Da Oger).

Urticaria

Presentation

- This can be acute or chronic (>6 weeks in duration).
- There can be multiple triggers such as foods, chemicals, medication, temperature changes and stress.
- Often it is difficult to identify an obvious cause.
- Enquire about any shortness of breath, facial swelling or tongue swelling, as these would be indications for a direct transfer to hospital via ambulance.

Often patients may present with a recurrent episode and term it to be an 'allergic reaction'.

A video or face-to-face consultation may be required to confirm the diagnosis.

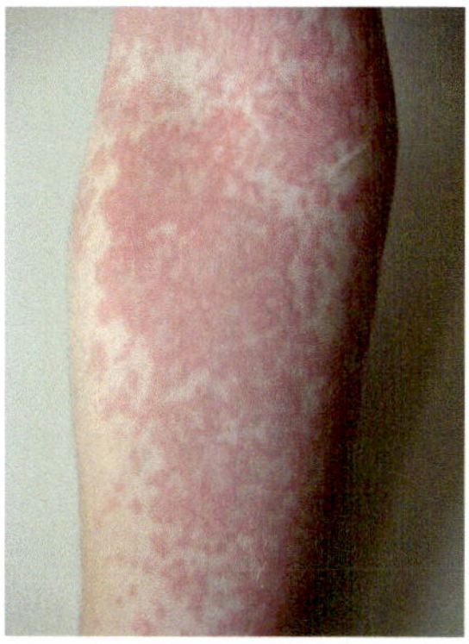

Fig. 17.18: Urticarial rash of the arm.

Reproduced from https://commons.wikimedia.org/wiki/File:EMminor2010.JPG under a CC BY-SA 3.0 licence (photo by James Heilman, MD).

Assessment

- It presents with raised, blanching, intensely pruritic hives and wheals anywhere on the body (*Fig. 17.18*).
- General observations will be normal and the patient will be well.

Management:

- This is based on controlling the excessive histamine response triggered by the cause; this includes oral chlorphenamine 4mg QDS × 7 days or fexofenadine 180mg once a day × 7 days.
- Severe urticaria or that which is unresponsive to oral antihistamines can be managed with oral prednisolone up to 20mg once a day × 5 days.
- Topical corticosteroids such as hydrocortisone 1% cream may also provide some relief from the pruritus.
- If there are features of anaphylaxis then the patient should be referred to ED via an emergency ambulance.

Varicella zoster (chickenpox)

Presentation

- This is caused by the herpes virus and results in a generalised vesicular (blistering) erythematous rash (*Fig. 17.19*).
- Patients are usually well; however, the rash can be intensely pruritic.

Chickenpox is a well-known viral skin condition and most people will be able to identify and diagnose the condition themselves. If there is any doubt, photographs or a video consultation should be enough to establish the diagnosis. In patients with no complications and where the diagnosis is obvious, telephone advice will usually suffice or signposting the patient to their pharmacist.

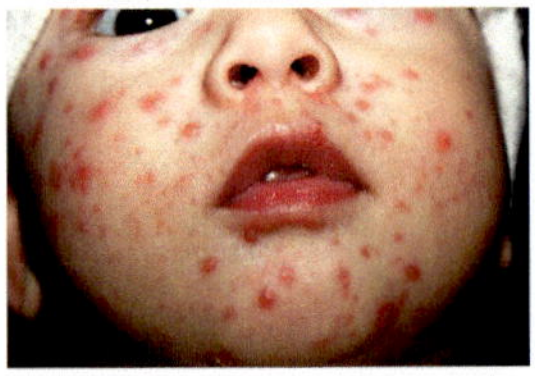

Fig. 17.19: Chickenpox rash.

Reproduced from https://commons.wikimedia.org/wiki/File:Vannkopper_chickenpox.JPG under a CC BY-SA 4.0 licence (photo by Øyvind Holmstad).

Management[12]

- It is self-limiting and the symptoms can be controlled with topical calamine lotion, oral antihistamines and paracetamol.
- Patients should be advised that the lesions are contagious until they become dry, and this can take 10–14 days to occur.
- Pregnant women who have been in contact with individuals who have had chickenpox should be offered serology testing; if they are at risk of infection then immunoglobulin protection should be offered.
- It is important to be aware of complications that can occur with varicella zoster; these include superimposed bacterial infections, meningitis, encephalitis, cerebellitis and pneumonitis.
- Ibuprofen should be avoided due to an increased risk of developing necrotising fasciitis.
- Patients with suspected complications should be referred to hospital immediately.

Varicose (stasis) eczema

Presentation and assessment

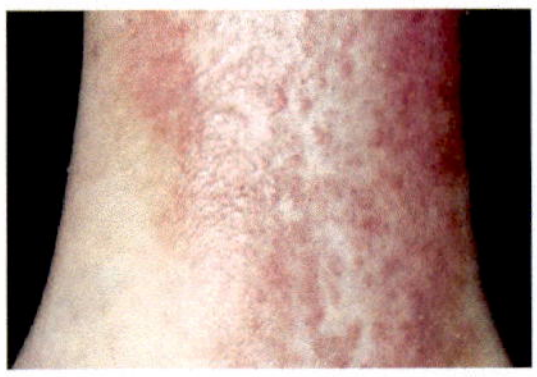

Fig. 17.20: Varicose eczema.

Reproduced from www.nhs.uk/conditions/varicose-eczema/ under an Open Government Licence.

- It is important to be able to differentiate skin changes which occur with varicose (stasis) eczema and cellulitis (*Fig. 17.20)*; often this can be done over the phone.
- Varicose or stasis eczema will have a protracted course and although the skin can appear erythematous and shiny as well as feeling warm, it will not be painful or tender.
- In those with varicose or stasis eczema, body temperature and observations will be within normal range.
- Inflammatory markers such as CRP will also be within normal range.

Differentiating between cellulitis and varicose eczema

Cellulitis	vs.	*Varicose eczema*
Quicker onset		Gradual onset
Erythema		Erythema
Shiny skin		Shiny skin
Warm to touch		Warm to touch
Painful		Painless
Tender		Non-tender

Management

- Varicose or stasis eczema is managed with the use of topical emollients and corticosteroids.

Summary for dermatology

- If necessary, examine the skin head to toe.
- Be aware of extra skin manifestations associated with some acute dermatological conditions.
- Prescriptions for topical corticosteroids should specify the duration of use.
- Mild cases of impetigo can resolve without treatment.
- The appearances of stasis eczema are similar to cellulitis.
- Koplik spots are pathognomonic of measles.
- The rash of meningococcal septicaemia develops peripherally.

References

1 Michael, Y. and Shaukat, N.M. (2021) *Erysipelas*. StatPearls. Available at: www.ncbi.nlm.nih.gov/books/NBK532247

2. NICE (updated 2018) *Lyme disease* [NG95]. Available at: www.nice.org.uk/guidance/ng95/chapter/recommendations

3. NHS (no date) *Hand, foot and mouth disease*. Available at: www.nhs.uk/conditions/hand-foot-mouth-disease/

4. NICE (revised 2024) *Hand foot and mouth disease* – Management. Available at: https://cks.nice.org.uk/hand-foot-and-mouth-disease

5. NICE (revised 2024) *Shingles* – Management. Available at: https://cks.nice.org.uk/shingles

6. British Association of Dermatologists (2021) *Impetigo*. Patient information leaflets. Available at: www.bad.org.uk/pils/impetigo/

7. NICE (revised 2024) *Impetigo*. Available at: https://cks.nice.org.uk/impetigo#!topicSummary

8. NHS (no date) *Measles*. Available at: www.nhs.uk/conditions/measles/

9. NICE (updated 2024) *Sepsis: recognition, diagnosis and early management* [NG51]. Available at: www.nice.org.uk/guidance/ng51

10. Staroselsky, A., Klieger-Grossmann, C., Garcia-Bournissen, F. and Koren, G. (2009) Exposure to fifth disease in pregnancy. *Can Fam Physician*, **55(12):** 1195–1198. Available at: www.ncbi.nlm.nih.gov/pmc/articles/PMC2793222/#:~:text=Parvovirus%20B19%20infection%20during%20pregnancy,fetalis%2C%20and%20even%20fetal%20demise.

11. NHS (no date) *Pityriasis rosea*. Available at: www.nhs.uk/conditions/pityriasis-rosea/

12. NICE (revised 2023) *Chickenpox* – Management. Available at: https://cks.nice.org.uk/chickenpox#!management

18

Chapter 18: **ENT**

ACUTE EAR CONDITIONS

"We have two ears and one mouth so we can listen twice as much as we speak."
Epictetus

Assessment of patients presenting with earache

Telephone

- There are several causes of earache and not all causes of earache will be due to infections.
- In some cases the pain may be originating from nearby structures such as the temporomandibular joint and causing referred pain to the ear.
- It is essential to ascertain a history of trauma or injudicious use of cotton buds, as these can cause prolonged earache and infections.
- Also one must not forget that overenthusiastic use of earphones and headphones with loud music can cause barotrauma.
- Mild infections are commonly viral in aetiology.
- Patients who are generally well can be reassured via telephone triage and directed to the pharmacist for analgesia and topical ear sprays such as Otocalm or EarCalm, with the proviso that the pain should settle within 7 days.

Face-to-face

A face-to-face assessment is recommended in the following circumstances:

- The presence of otorrhoea (discharge)
- The presence of a high temperature
- The presence of facial swelling
- Symptoms for more than 72 hours and these are progressive in nature
- There is doubt about the aetiology of the earache or if the patient is generally unwell.

Herpes zoster can present with earache, so always look into the ear for the presence of vesicles.

If the cause is not obvious consider referred pain from the temporomandibular joint, teeth or intra-oral pathology.

Palpate the neck for any swellings such as reactive cervical lymphadenopathy associated with infections.

Red flag features for earache

- Persistent earache
- Dysphagia
- Dysphonia
- Weight loss
- Visual symptoms
- In the elderly consider temporal arteritis

Otitis externa

Presentation

- Pain will be the most common presenting feature.
- Patients may also complain of a discharge.
- Oedema of the ear canal and the presence of a discharge will affect hearing.
- Insertion of foreign bodies such as cotton buds is a common precursor.

Patients with mild symptoms can be advised to take appropriate analgesia and signposted to their local pharmacist for over-the-counter topical ear drops. However, if there is a discharge or the patient is generally unwell a face-to-face assessment may be required.

Also, ear drops will be of limited value in patients who have a discharge.

Assessment

- Most patients will be generally well with normal observations.
- When assessing the ear it is important to assess the mastoid process to rule out mastoiditis.
- Inflammation of the ear canal will be evident (*Fig 18.1*), especially when compared to the contralateral ear; however, the tympanic membrane will appear normal (dull or pearly grey in colour; see *Fig. 18.2*).

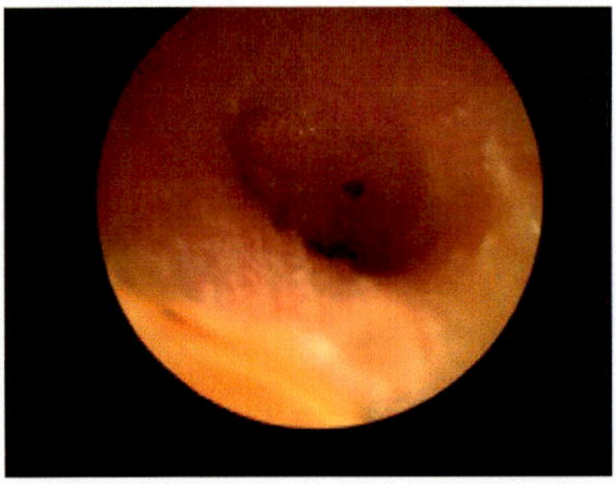

Fig. 18.1: Otitis externa with a perforation of the tympanic membrane.

Reproduced from http://sydneyentclinic.com/sean-flanagan/ courtesy of Dr Sean Flanagan, Sydney ENT Clinic.

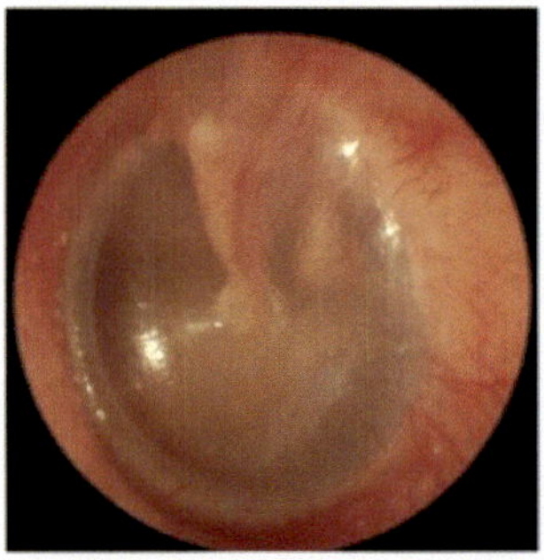

Fig. 18.2: A normal tympanic membrane.

Reproduced from http://sydneyentclinic.com/sean-flanagan/ courtesy of Dr Sean Flanagan, Sydney ENT Clinic.

Management[1]

- Patients should be advised to mitigate against causative factors such as swimming, and to avoid cotton buds at all costs.
- Mild cases can be managed with topical agents available from the pharmacy such as Otocalm or EarCalm.
- Alternative topical agents available on prescription include Otomize spray, Sofradex or Gentisone ear drops.
- Appropriate oral analgesia should be advised.
- Patients in whom symptoms and signs suggest a more severe infection, or if the status of the tympanic membrane cannot be confirmed, should be prescribed oral antibiotics such as flucloxacillin 250–500mg QDS × 7 days or clarithromycin 250–500mg BD × 7 days.
- A macrolide antibiotic such as clarithromycin will cover bacterial organisms responsible for otitis externa and otitis media and would be the antibiotic of choice if there is doubt regarding which condition the patient has, or if a face-to-face assessment is not possible.
- Patients may also benefit from microsuction to remove any discharge and debris, although this should be postponed until the infection is under control.
- Patients presenting with recurrent otitis externa may benefit from having swabs taken to isolate atypical causative organisms such as *Pseudomonas* and *Candida* and to determine their sensitivities to antimicrobials. If there is involvement of the outer ear and cartilage, then this is termed perichondritis. It is usually the result of an infected piercing and should be treated with oral ciprofloxacin and not flucloxacillin, as the causative organism is usually *Pseudomonas*.
- Systemically unwell patients should be referred to the on-call ear, nose and throat (ENT) team.

Otitis media

Presentation

- Patients will usually complain of pain in the ear; this will be deep-seated, often made worse by biting down.
- There may be a discharge, which may be bloodstained.
- Hearing will be affected.
- The patient may have a high temperature.

Most infective cases are of viral origin, and patients with mild symptoms of less than 72 hours' duration can be managed over the phone and advised to take appropriate analgesia.

The presence of systemic or prolonged symptoms warrants a physical assessment to determine the severity and cause of the earache.

Assessment[1]

- It is uncommon for the patient to be systemically unwell.
- Again, it is important to examine the mastoid process and rule out mastoiditis.
- The tympanic membrane will be hyperaemic, bulging and inflamed (*Fig. 18.3*).
- The ear canal may also be inflamed, indicating concomitant otitis externa.

Management[2],[3]

- Most cases tend to be viral and it is appropriate to wait 72 hours before initiating antibiotic treatment in systemically well patients.
- In such cases reassurance and analgesia should suffice; however, you can consider a delayed prescription handed to the patient and advise if symptoms do not improve in 72 hours or symptoms worsen or additional features develop, such as a discharge, then the patient should start the antibiotics. This can help reassure the patient that they have something to start if the infection does not settle or if it progresses.
- Always advise the patient that if they have any concerns despite starting antibiotics, to seek medical attention.
- For patients who have a discharge, prolonged symptoms or if a bacterial infection is suspected, the antibiotics of choice are amoxicillin 250–500mg TDS × 7 days or a macrolide such as clarithromycin 250–500mg BD × 7 days.
- Systemically unwell patients or those suspected of having or being at risk of sepsis should be referred to the on-call ENT team.
- Patients presenting with recurrent otitis media or a persistent discharge may benefit from having swabs taken to isolate causative organisms and determining sensitivities to antimicrobials.

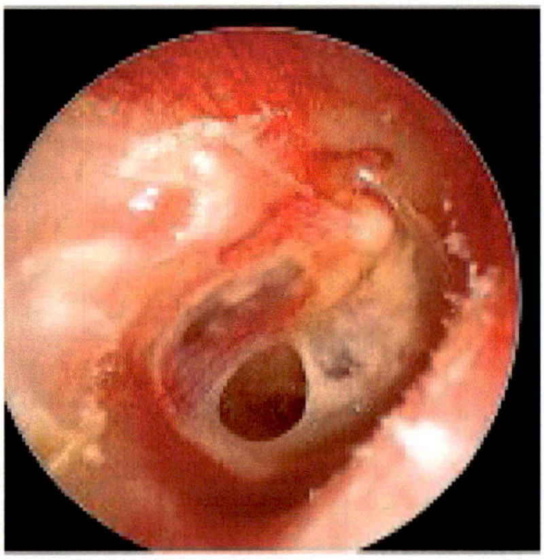

Fig. 18.3: Otitis media with a perforation of the tympanic membrane.

Reproduced from http://sydneyentclinic.com/sean-flanagan/ courtesy of Dr Sean Flanagan, Sydney ENT Clinic.

Otitis media with effusion (glue ear)

Presentation

- Patients with glue ear will usually be pain-free due to the absence of acute inflammation.
- Hearing loss is a common presenting feature, with patients often suspecting earwax to be the cause.
- It is thought 50% of cases follow an episode of acute otitis media, resulting in the accumulation of fluid in the middle ear[4].
- It is the most common cause of hearing impairment in children and predisposing conditions include cleft lip or palate, cystic fibrosis and allergic rhinitis[4].

Assessment

- A face-to-face assessment is required to confirm the diagnosis and to rule out other causes of impaired hearing.
- On examination the tympanic membrane will appear dull and retracted.

- There will be a visible fluid level behind the tympanic membrane as well as trapped air bubbles (*Fig. 18.4*).

Management

- Spontaneous resolution will occur in the majority of cases; however, this can take up to 3 months.
- If there is evidence of an infection, then this should be treated with oral antibiotics.
- Analgesia, along with oral decongestants such as pseudoephedrine, may help although the evidence is scant.
- Steroid nasal sprays, steam and menthol inhalation may also help to relieve nasal and Eustachian tube congestion.
- Chronic effusions may require grommets; more so in children, where any associated deafness can affect speech development. In such cases an outpatient referral to the ENT surgeons is warranted.

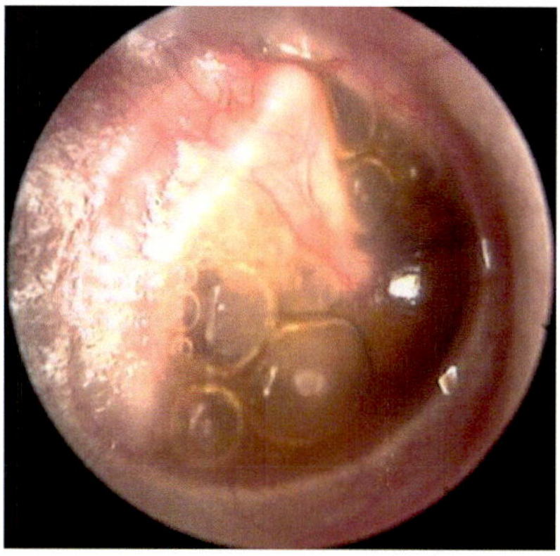

Fig. 18.4: Otitis media with an effusion.

Reproduced from http://sydneyentclinic.com/sean-flanagan/ courtesy of Dr Sean Flanagan, Sydney ENT Clinic.

Eustachian tube dysfunction

Presentation

- This can be acute, as seen in upper respiratory tract infections and following air travel, or chronic, as is the case with glue ear.
- Patients will present with decreased hearing, tinnitus and occasionally pain.

Assessment

- The patient will be well and general observations will be normal.
- The tympanic membrane on the affected side will appear dull and retracted.
- It may appear hyperaemic if the underlying condition has caused inflammation.
- There may be fluid in the middle ear, indicating blockage of the Eustachian tube.

Management

- This is based on treating the underlying cause and allowing the pressure changes in the Eustachian tube to return to normal.
- Occasionally a corticosteroid nasal spray and oral pseudoephedrine may help to alleviate congestion in the tubes and hasten recovery.

Mastoiditis

Presentation

- Mastoiditis commonly affects children.
- It may present on its own or with accompanying otitis media.

Assessment

- Mastoiditis should always be excluded when a patient presents with ear or jaw pain.
- Hence when examining the ear it is good practice to make a habit of examining the mastoid process.
- The patient (and especially children) may be generally unwell with a pyrexia and tachycardia.
- Characteristically the mastoid bone is inflamed, swollen and tender.

Management

- Adult patients should be started on co-amoxiclav 625mg TDS × 7 days or a macrolide such as clarithromycin 500mg BD × 7 days.
- Systemically unwell patients and children with mastoiditis should be referred to the on-call ENT team.

Labyrinthitis and acute vestibular neuritis

Presentation

- When a patient complains of 'dizziness', it is important to differentiate whether this is vertigo or a feeling of light-headedness, as the causes of both are very different.
- Light-headedness can be caused by a number of factors such as hypotension, dehydration, low blood glucose levels, alcohol or drug intoxication, and anxiety.
- Vertigo refers to a sensation of one's surroundings spinning, resulting in impaired balance and coordination.
- The two most common causes of vertigo are acute vestibular neuritis (AVN), due to inflammation of the vestibular ganglion, and labyrinthitis, due to inflammation of the labyrinth.
- Both these structures sit within the inner ear.
- Inflammation causes vertigo, nausea, vomiting, hearing loss, tinnitus and loss of balance.
- Onset tends to be sudden and can be from viral infections, head injuries, medication and extreme stress.

Patients who have mild vertigo and those where the cause is suspected to be viral can be managed over the phone. Promethazine and cinnarizine, both of which are antihistamines and are available over the counter, can help with mild symptoms; alternatively a prescription can be issued remotely, provided a tight safety-net has been applied.

Otherwise a face-to-face assessment is required and occasionally a home visit if the patient is unable to get to a clinic.

Assessment

- Head movements will make the symptoms worse.
- Speech, limb and cranial nerve examinations will be within normal limits.
- Romberg's test will be negative; however, nystagmus may be present.
- The presence of ataxia, dysarthria and dysdiadochokinesis indicate a cerebellar cause such as a cerebellar stroke, and a referral to the on-call medical team is warranted.

Management

- In the vast majority of cases the inflammation is caused by a viral infection and spontaneous resolution is expected within 7–14 days.
- Oral or buccal prochlorperazine will assist in controlling symptoms.
- Alternative agents are betahistine, cinnarizine, promethazine and cyclizine.
- Rarely, IM medication may be required.
- Symptoms lasting for more than 14 days warrant further investigations.

Summary for acute ear conditions

- Not all ear pain is due to an infection; also consider referred pain.
- In patients presenting with ear pain always perform a full examination, checking observations to rule out sepsis and examining the mastoid process.
- Mild ear infections are viral in origin and can be managed with observation and analgesia for the first 72 hours.

References

1. BNF (no date) *Ear* – Treatment summary. Available at: https://bnf.nice.org.uk/treatment-summary/ear.html

2. NICE (updated 2022) *Otitis media (acute): antimicrobial prescribing* [NG91]. Available at: www.nice.org.uk/guidance/ng91/chapter/Recommendations#managing-acute-otitis-media

3. Harmes, K.M., Blackwood, R.A., Burrows, H.L. *et al.* (2013) Otitis media: diagnosis and treatment. *American Family Physician*, **88(7):** 435–440.

4. NICE (revised 2023) *Otitis media with effusion*. Available at: https://cks.nice.org.uk/topics/otitis-media-with-effusion/

ACUTE NASAL PROBLEMS

"It's not how you pick your nose, it's where you put that booger that counts."
Tré Cool

Assessment of patients presenting with acute nasal problems

Telephone

- Although a detailed history can be taken over the phone, most patients with an acute nasal problem will require a face-to-face appointment; an exception will be rhinitis, which can be managed with telephone advice and signposting to the pharmacy.
- Another exception may also be acute sinusitis, especially if this is recurrent and patients already have a management plan in place. As a result they may be calling to request a prescription for antibiotics.

Face-to-face

- All patients with active epistaxis or nasal trauma should have their general observations assessed and documented.

Findings prior to and after removal of a foreign body should be documented.

Epistaxis

Presentation

- Always ask about common causes such as trauma and picking at the nose (surprisingly common amongst young children who present with epistaxis, although denial of this is just as common).
- Epistaxis is also relatively common in the elderly and those on anticoagulant therapy; however, often a cause is not found.
- Patients should be advised to apply constant pressure to the bottom third of the nose for at least 15 minutes.

If this does not stop the bleeding then a referral to ED or an urgent treatment centre is warranted for a face-to-face assessment.

Assessment

- It is important to check basic observations, as hypertension can be a contributing factor.
- Checking vital signs will also assist in determining the extent of blood loss.
- The use of additional lighting and a nasal speculum may help to identify the source of bleeding.

- Advise the patient to sit upright to prevent swallowing of blood.

Management[1],[2]

- Most occurrences cease with constant pressure applied to the bottom third of the nose for 15 minutes.
- Applying pressure to the nasal bones will not stop the bleeding.
- Once the bleeding has stopped, the patient should be advised to avoid picking or blowing the nose.
- Hot foods, showers or baths should be avoided for 48 hours.
- Naseptin cream or mupirocin ointment applied three times a day for 10 days can help prevent nasal infections and aid the healing of any abrasions and vestibulitis.
- If the source of bleeding is seen and provided adequate resources are available, cauterisation can be attempted.
- Patients in whom bleeding has failed to settle with the above measures should be referred to the local ED for tamponade.
- Patients presenting with a large amount of blood loss or signs to suggest this (e.g. tachycardia, hypotension) should be referred to the ED.
- Elderly patients and those on anticoagulants are at increased risk of heavy bleeding, especially from the posterior cavity. For these reasons consider an early referral to ED for nasal tamponade.

Intranasal foreign bodies

Presentation

- More often than not this will be a child.

Management

- Removal can be attempted; however, it is important to have the appropriate equipment.
- Portable ENT kits are available and it is always helpful to have one as part of a doctor's bag.
- It is important to document your examination findings before and after removal.
- Any failed attempts should be referred to the ED or local ENT team on call.

Nasal trauma

Presentation

- Patients with all but mild nasal trauma should be referred for a face-to-face assessment.

Assessment

- Always check basic observations, as this will assist in determining the extent of blood loss or the possibility of additional injuries.

- It is important to ensure there is no septal haematoma, as this can cause destruction of the nasal cartilage and result in permanent deformity.
- Examine inside the nasal passages using an otoscope and a nasal speculum, observing for a septal haematoma and any sources of bleeding.
- Document your findings, including the absence of any complications.

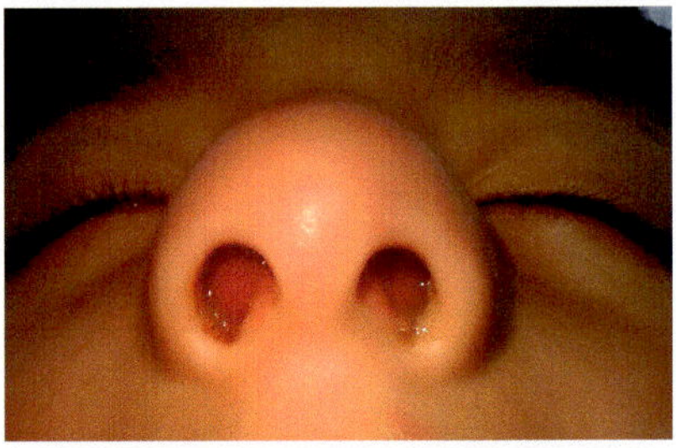

Fig. 18.5: A nasal septal haematoma in an 8-year-old boy following facial trauma.

Management[3]

- Minor trauma can be managed with reassurance, ice packs to reduce swelling and oral analgesia.
- If there is a visible deformity after 10 days the patient should be advised to see their own GP, as a routine outpatient referral to the ENT surgeons may be required.
- If there is a gross deformity, a septal haematoma or if the patient presents with trouble breathing, refer immediately to the on-call ENT team.

Rhinitis

Presentation

- There are several different types including seasonal, allergic, perennial and vasomotor.
- Often the diagnosis can be made over the phone.
- Patients will be systemically well.
- Allergic rhinitis may be associated with allergic conjunctivitis.
- Vasomotor rhinitis is more common in the elderly and usually occurs when there is a change in ambient temperature; for example, moving from a warm to a cold room, or when about to eat a hot meal.

Assessment

- A face-to-face assessment is rarely required unless there are red flag features such as unilateral persistent nasal discharge or a bloodstained discharge.
- Examination of the nasal passages will reveal a congested and hyperaemic mucosal lining.
- There may be hypertrophy of the nasal turbinates.
- In some cases chronic nasal polyps may have developed.

Management

- Oral antihistamines can be used for most forms of rhinitis with varying efficacy; these include cetirizine 10mg once daily and loratadine 10mg once daily, both of which are available to purchase from the pharmacy.

- Topical corticosteroids also help, e.g. beclomethasone nasal spray twice daily × 4 weeks. Again this is available to purchase from the pharmacy.
- Vasomotor rhinitis responds to topical ipratropium bromide spray.

Nasal furuncle

Presentation

- This is a boil of the face which can rapidly cause cellulitis.
- Pain, swelling and redness of the area are the most common presenting features.

In generally well patients a video consultation may suffice, especially if the patient is able to check their own vital signs. If this is not possible or the patient appears to be unwell, a face-to-face assessment should be arranged.

Assessment

- Vital signs should be measured.
- The affected area will be swollen, erythematous and tender.
- The extent of erythema and swelling should be documented.

Management

- Mild cases can be treated with oral antibiotics such as flucloxacillin or clarithromycin.
- Patients who are acutely unwell should be referred to the on-call ENT team.

Acute sinusitis

Presentation

- This presents with a headache and facial pain.
- Invariably the maxillary sinuses or, less commonly, the frontal sinuses are affected.
- There may be an associated thick nasal discharge, often described in various forms and a multitude of bright colours.
- Patients will often sound congested, with a nasal twang to their voice.
- The pain tends to be worse on flexing the neck forwards.
- Patients with mild and early symptoms can be referred to their local pharmacist, as most cases tend to be viral in origin and conservative measures will suffice.

A video consultation may help in assessing the patient; however, patients who are systemically unwell, have severe symptoms or have facial swelling should have a face-to-face assessment.

Assessment

- There will be facial tenderness.
- There may be facial swelling over the affected areas.
- The patient may be systemically unwell so it is important to check observations.
- Consider the possibility of referred pain from other structures such as the teeth.

Management[4]

- Most cases tend to be viral and settle with over-the-counter medication such as oral analgesics and anti-inflammatories.
- Nasal and oral decongestants will help, along with steam and menthol vapour inhalation.
- Patients can be referred to their pharmacist under the Pharmacy First scheme (in England) for assessment and, if needed, antibiotics.
- Prolonged cases (>10 days) or those associated with systemic symptoms should be managed with oral antibiotics such as amoxicillin 250–500mg TDS × 5–7 days or a macrolide such as clarithromycin 250–500mg BD × 5–7 days or a tetracycline such as doxycycline.
- If the patient is systemically unwell or has complications such as orbital cellulitis, they should be referred to ED or the on-call ENT surgeons.

Red flag features in patients with nasal or sinus problems

Patients presenting with recurrent sinusitis or a persistent unilateral nasal or bloodstained discharge should be advised to see their GP immediately to consider investigations to rule out sinister pathology.

Summary for acute nasal problems

- Checking observations will assist in determining the extent of any blood loss with nasal trauma.
- A septal haematoma must be ruled out with acute nasal injuries.
- Patients presenting with recurrent sinusitis or a persistent unilateral nasal or bloodstained discharge should be advised to see their GP immediately to consider investigations to rule out sinister pathology.

References

1. NICE (2019) *Epistaxis (nosebleeds)*. Available at: https://cks.nice.org.uk/topics/epistaxis-nosebleeds

2. Kucik, C.J. and Clenney, T. (2005) Management of epistaxis. *American Family Physician*, **71(2):** 305–311.

3. Razavi, A., Farboud, A., Skinner, R. and Saw, K. (2014) Acute nasal injury. *BMJ*, **349:** g6537. Available at: https://doi.org/10.1136/bmj.g6537

4. Falagas, M.E., Giannopoulou, K.P., Vardakas, K.Z. *et al.* (2008) Comparison of antibiotics with placebo for treatment of acute sinusitis: a meta-analysis of randomised controlled trials. *Lancet Infectious Diseases*, **8(9):** 543–552.

ACUTE THROAT PROBLEMS

"It's better to keep your mouth shut and appear stupid than open it and remove all doubt."
Mark Twain

Assessment of patients presenting with a sore throat

Telephone

- Most patients who present with a sore throat can be assessed over the telephone.
- The most common cause of an acute sore throat is usually a viral infection which is benign and self-limiting.
- Supportive measures are required and patients can be given advice over the telephone as well as being directed to their pharmacist.

Face-to-face

Face-to-face assessment would be required in the following situations:

- Patients with systemic symptoms and to rule out sepsis.
- To identify any conditions which will require hospital admission, e.g. quinsy.
- Patients who are unable to swallow.
- Patients claiming to have pustules or an exudate at the back of their throat.

Patients have become quite adept at 'examining' their own throat and they will often self-declare the presence of 'white spots' on their 'tonsils'; their presence does not always indicate a bacterial infection, as is the case with an Epstein–Barr virus (EBV) infection; however, it can indicate a streptococcal infection, thereby justifying a request for oral antibiotics. On such occasions a photograph or a video consultation may help.

If assessing the patient face-to-face, always palpate the neck for any swellings such as reactive cervical lymphadenopathy associated with infections.

Glandular fever (infectious mononucleosis)

Presentation

- Glandular fever is a viral infection caused by EBV, which mainly affects teenagers and young adults.
- It is characterised by a sore throat, high temperature, swollen neck glands, malaise and fatigue.
- Headaches and abdominal pain may also be present.
- Some patients may also have a rash.

A face-to-face assessment is usually required to assess patients with suspected glandular fever due to the presence of systemic features.

Assessment

Check for:

- A high temperature and tachycardia – patients may be systemically unwell.
- Enlarged tonsils with bilateral exudates.
- Cervical lymphadenopathy, with the lymph nodes being smooth, homogeneous and tender.
- Splenomegaly via an abdominal examination, because it is also a notable feature.
- A blanching maculopapular rash on the torso – although this is not always present.

Management

- Management should be supportive, as the causative agent is a virus and the condition is self-limiting.
- Use oral rehydration, analgesia, anaesthetic lozenges and anaesthetic throat sprays.
- In protracted cases, blood tests for serology may be helpful in confirming the diagnosis and avoiding the need for unnecessary antibiotics, as early features can often mimic acute bacterial tonsillitis.
- If a secondary bacterial infection is suspected, phenoxymethylpenicillin or a macrolide such as clarithromycin are the antibiotics of choice. Avoid amoxicillin and ampicillin because they can cause a rash in patients who have active glandular fever.
- Complications such as pericarditis and rupture of the spleen are rare; however, if these are suspected or the patient is systemically unwell, dehydrated or jaundiced, then referral to the on-call medical team should be arranged.

Red flag features in patients with glandular fever

- Systemically unwell
- Pericarditis: chest pain, dyspnoea, ECG changes
- Splenic rupture: severe abdominal pain, hypovolaemic shock, splenic tenderness

Laryngitis

Presentation

- Typically, dysphonia (hoarse voice) or atypically, aphonia (complete loss of voice).
- Low-grade pyrexia and a sore throat are also common.

A face-to-face assessment is rarely required because most cases of laryngitis cause dysphonia (and not aphonia). The diagnosis is usually clear over the phone and can be managed with conservative measures.

Assessment

- Dysphonia will be apparent on taking a history.
- Occasionally assessment may require a lot of patience and occasionally a pen and paper or improvised sign language, if the patient is struggling to articulate a verbal history.

- Reassuringly most cases are due to a viral infection or overexertion of the vocal cords (often seen in teachers of an unruly class at school).

Management

- This is centred on resting the voice, pain relief and oral anti-inflammatory medication such as ibuprofen.
- Fluids and steam inhalation may help.
- Evidence suggests that antibiotics have no benefit in improving outcome, but may improve subjective symptoms[1].

Persistent dysphonia, especially in the elderly or patients with a history of tobacco consumption, requires investigation and patients may require a flexible nasolaryngoscopy to rule out sinister pathology.

Neck swellings

- **Acute neck swellings** without any other symptoms are rarely seen in an urgent care setting, because the onset of most neck swellings tends to be insidious. In nearly all cases a face-to-face assessment will be required to assess the swelling.
- **Acute thyroid swellings** are rare in an urgent primary care setting and the most common cause of thyroid swellings is a goitre. This tends to be of gradual onset and the patient's presentation may have been triggered by anxieties regarding sinister medical conditions. Reassurance and referral back to the patient's GP will usually suffice.
- **Cervical lymphadenopathy** is commonly due to viral infections, with common culprits being the Epstein–Barr virus (infectious mononucleosis) or the mumps virus; however, often it will be due to a non-specific viral infection. Clinical examination reveals smooth, homogeneous, tender lymphadenopathy, usually of the anterior cervical chain nodes. Management is conservative because self-resolution is expected.
- **Parotid gland swellings**, which are acute and painful in the young, are due to viruses, e.g. mumps (can result in orchitis in boys and subfertility in men). Treatment is based on reassurance, hydration, analgesia and appropriate safety-netting. Unilateral swellings, especially in the elderly, should be investigated with appropriate imaging – an ultrasound scan would be an appropriate first-line examination.
- **Submandibular gland swellings** are commonly due to infection or a stone blocking the salivary duct. Treatment is based on encouraging salivation by ingesting sour substances and massage of the submandibular gland. Antibiotics such as co-amoxiclav 625mg TDS × 7 days or clarithromycin 500mg BD × 7 days can be used to treat suspected bacterial infections.

Any swelling lasting for more than two weeks or of a progressive nature warrants further investigation such as ultrasound imaging, or an urgent outpatient referral to the ENT surgeons.

Pharyngitis

Presentation

- A detailed history can be taken over the telephone.
- Commonly caused by a viral infection and therefore the majority of cases tend to be benign and self-limiting.

A video consultation may assist in reassuring the patient if anxiety levels are high. However, if a video consultation will not suffice, or if the patient is systemically unwell, or at high risk of developing complications (e.g. immunocompromised), or the history is unclear, then a face-to-face assessment is warranted.

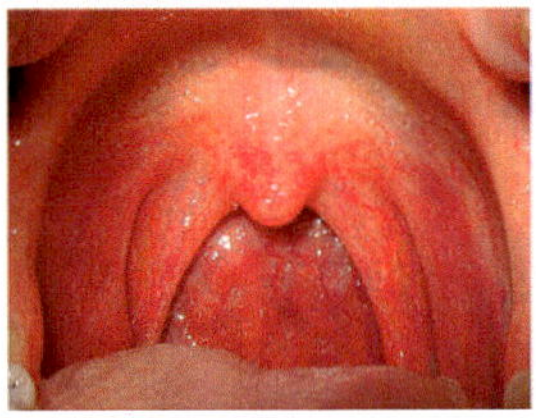

Fig 18.6: Acute viral pharyngitis.

Reproduced from https://commons.wikimedia.org/wiki/File:Pharyngitis.jpg under a CC BY-SA 2.5 licence (photo by Dake).

Assessment

- If a physical examination is undertaken, general observations will usually be within normal limits, although low-grade pyrexia may be present.
- On inspection the pharynx will appear inflamed (*Fig. 18.6*); however, the tonsillar pillars will be spared or will be quiescent.
- Inflammation of the pharynx may be severe and occasionally an exudate may be present.

Management

- A request for antibiotics will usually follow when someone presents with a sore throat, and a skilled clinician will explain patiently that no amount of antibiotics will treat a viral infection!
- The mainstay of treatment will be reassurance, lozenges (e.g. Strepsils, Merocaine and Tyrozets), topical anaesthetic sprays (e.g. Difflam), fluids and analgesia (paracetamol, ibuprofen)[2].
- Advising the patient that the lozenges will have an antiseptic and anaesthetic in them may help to reassure patients, especially those who are keen to have an antibiotic on prescription.
- Providing a delayed prescription for antibiotics specifying an approximate timeframe (e.g. 72hrs) before using can also help relieve patient anxiety.
- Approximately 85% of viral throat infections last 7–10 days, and this should be relayed to the patient. Symptoms usually peak around day 4–5, which is commonly when most patients present.
- If the patient has symptoms lasting more than 7 days, is generally unwell or has suspected bacterial pharyngitis (widespread severe inflammation with an exudate), swabs can be taken to determine the causative organism. However, the most common cause of bacterial pharyngitis is *Streptococcus* which is sensitive to penicillin and macrolide antibiotics, so it is reasonable to prescribe penicillin V 250–500mg QDS × 10 days or clarithromycin 500mg BD × 7 days.
- Systemically unwell patients, or those with suspected sepsis or who are unable to swallow, should be admitted to hospital.

The CENTOR criteria[3] can be applied to assist in determining if antibiotics should be prescribed:

Cough, Exudate, Nodes (tender and enlarged), Temperature; score 1 for the presence of each of these parameters.

A score of 0, 1 or 2 is associated with a 3–17% likelihood of isolating *Streptococcus*; hence antibiotics are usually not warranted. A score of 3 or 4 is thought to be associated with a 32–56% likelihood of isolating *Streptococcus*.

The Modified CENTOR criteria also take into account a patient's age; if the patient is aged under 15 years add 1 point, if the patient is aged over 44 years subtract 1 point.

Quinsy

Presentation

- Can occur quite suddenly and without warning; however, more often than not it will be preceded by bacterial tonsillitis; patients may already be on antibiotics.

Anyone who is suspected of having quinsy should be assessed face-to-face to establish the diagnosis; occasionally this can be undertaken via video consultation, provided the clinician is confident they can visualise the pharynx and tonsils clearly.

Assessment

- The patient is unable to swallow anything, including their own saliva.
- They may also be systemically unwell with pyrexia, tachycardia and hypotension.
- Always check the capillary blood glucose because oral intake will inevitably have been reduced and hypoglycaemia can occur as a result.
- Visual examination may be limited due to pain and an inability to open the mouth fully.

Management

- Once seen (*Fig. 18.7*), quinsy is unmistakeable.
- Once established, quinsy will require surgical intervention and a referral to the on-call ENT team is mandatory.
- If oral analgesia cannot be taken then rectal analgesia should be considered whilst arranging a transfer to hospital.
- The patient will require IV antibiotics and IV rehydration and if possible IV access should be obtained.
- For systemically unwell patients consider an ambulance transfer to hospital.

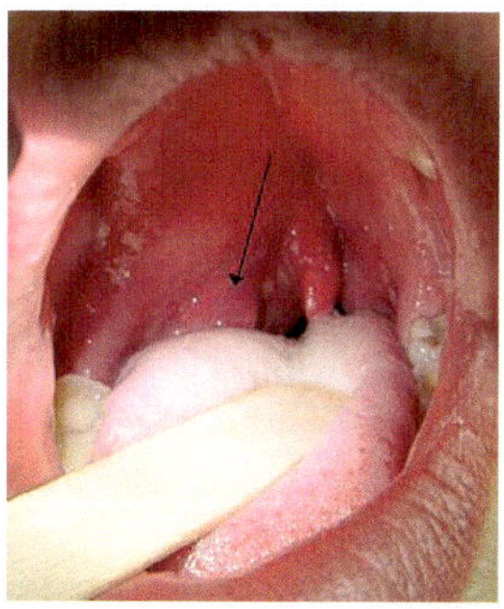

Fig. 18.7: A right-sided peri-tonsillar abscess or quinsy.

Scarlet fever

Presentation

- This is a bacterial infection caused by Group A *Streptococcus* (*S. pyogenes*); see also the section on Invasive Group A *Streptococcus* infections in *Chapter 22*.
- Children and adolescents are commonly affected.
- Initial features will include a sore throat and a high temperature; a rash follows a few days later.

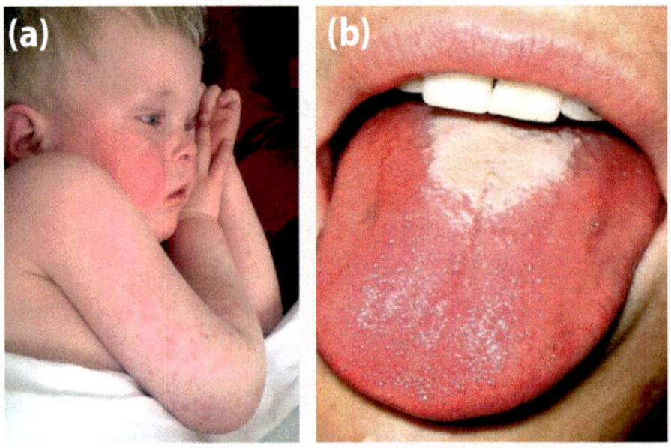

Fig. 18.8: (a) The rash of scarlet fever; (b) 'strawberry tongue'.

A face-to-face assessment is recommended due to the multiple sites involved and the difficulty in assessing rashes over the phone.

Assessment

- Patients may appear generally unwell.
- The rash will be most prominent on the chest and back, although the limbs can also be affected (*Fig. 18.8a*). Typically the rash will be erythematous, blanching and maculopapular in nature.
- The pharynx and tonsillar pillars will be inflamed and there may be a bilateral exudate.
- Characteristically the tongue will be inflamed and swollen with a white exudate, often being referred to as a 'strawberry tongue' (*Fig. 18.8b*).

Management

Scarlet fever is a notifiable disease in the UK and any suspected or confirmed cases should be notified to the local health protection team[4].

- Scarlet fever should be treated with antibiotics:
  - first-line is phenoxymethylpenicillin 500mg QDS × 10 days
  - if this is not tolerated then give amoxicillin 500mg TDS × 10 days
  - give azithromycin 500mg OD × 5 days to patients who are allergic to penicillin.
- Patients who are systemically unwell or unable to swallow oral antibiotics should be referred to the on-call medical team.

Tonsillitis

Presentation

- Patients with a sore throat will claim to have tonsillitis, only to be dumbfounded when you reassure them it is a viral infection and it will settle without antibiotics. Careful use of online images of true tonsillitis (*Fig. 18.9*) can help reassure the patient that they do not have life-threatening tonsillitis.
- However, some patients may be prone to recurrent tonsillitis and will wear this like a badge of honour.

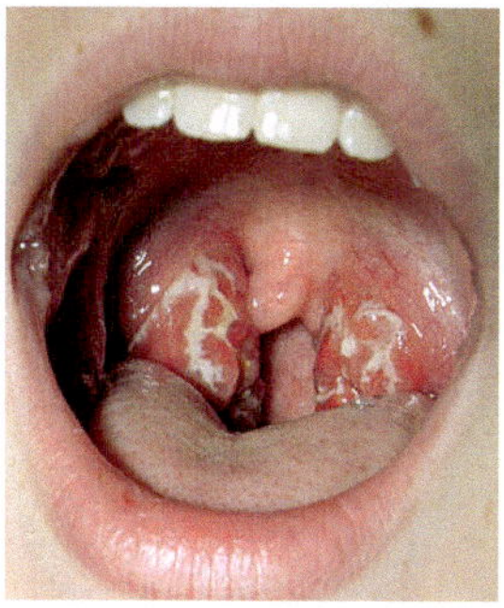

Fig. 18.9: Acute bacterial tonsillitis.

Reproduced from https://commons.wikimedia.org/wiki/File:IDApp.JPG under a CC BY-SA 4.0 licence (photo by Doc James).

A video consultation and occasional photos may be enough to establish the diagnosis of tonsillitis; however, if this is not possible, if there is high patient anxiety or a suspicion of possible complications such as quinsy, a face-to-face consultation should be arranged.

Assessment

- The tonsils will be enlarged and inflamed and there may be an exudate covering the tonsillar pillars.
- A general examination is important to ensure the patient is systemically well and to eliminate the possibility of sepsis.
- It is important to assess swallowing, because if this is not possible the patient will be at risk of dehydration and will also be unable to take oral antibiotics.

Management

- Although most cases of tonsillitis are viral, there may be justification in starting antibiotics. If the patient is systemically unwell or there is an exudate (bear in mind infectious mononucleosis may also present with bilateral exudates), then antibiotics may be prescribed.
- If a streptococcal infection is confirmed via throat swabs (usually not possible in an OOH setting) or suspected, then antibiotics are warranted[5].
- The following options are available:
  - penicillin V 500mg QDS × 10 days
  - clarithromycin 500mg BD × 10 days
  - erythromycin 500mg QDS × 10 days
- Consider prescribing suspensions as these are easier to swallow.
- The patient should take regular oral analgesia.
- Anaesthetic sprays and lozenges will also help.
- Emphasise the importance of keeping well hydrated.
- Advise the patient that they should see an improvement in 5 days; if this does not occur or symptoms worsen or if there are any concerns, then medical attention should be sought.
- Needless to say, this advice should be documented in the patient's clinical records.
- Systemically unwell patients, those with suspected sepsis, or those who are unable to swallow should be admitted to hospital.

Red flag features of acute sore throat indicating referral to hospital

- Systemically unwell
- Unable to swallow
- Dehydrated or at risk of dehydration
- Has quinsy

Summary for acute throat problems

- Most causes of a sore throat are viral. The CENTOR or Modified CENTOR criteria can be used to determine the need for antibiotics.
- Patients presenting with tonsillitis should be referred to hospital if they are systemically unwell, unable to swallow or have quinsy.
- Scarlet fever is a notifiable disease in the UK.
- Secondary bacterial infections can occur in glandular fever and antibiotics may be warranted; however, amoxicillin and ampicillin should be avoided because they can cause a rash in patients who have glandular fever.

References

1. Reveiz, L. (monitoring editor), Cardona, A.F. and Cochrane Acute Respiratory Infections Group (2015) Antibiotics for acute laryngitis in adults. *Cochrane Database Syst Rev*, **2015(5):** CD004783. Available at: www.ncbi.nlm.nih.gov/pmc/articles/PMC6486127/

2. NICE (2018) *Sore throat (acute): antimicrobial prescribing* [NG84]. Available at: www.nice.org.uk/guidance/ng84

3. Centor, R.M., Witherspoon, J.M., Dalton, H.P. *et al.* (1981) The diagnosis of strep throat in adults in the emergency room. *Med Decis Making,* **1**: 239–46.

4. NICE (revised 2024) *Scarlet fever* – Management. Available at: https://cks.nice.org.uk/scarlet-fever#!scenario

5. BMJ Best Practice (updated 2024) *Tonsillitis*. Available at: https://bestpractice.bmj.com/topics/en-gb/598

ACUTE DENTAL PROBLEMS

*"Some tortures are physical and some are mental,
but the one that is both, is dental."*
Ogden Nash

General assessment of patients presenting with dental problems

Telephone

- When a patient presents with suspected dental problems, make them aware that you are not a qualified dentist (unless of course you are a qualified dentist!).
- Most parts of the UK will have an OOH dental service commissioned by the NHS to provide emergency dental advice and treatment.
- Patients can usually be referred to their own or an emergency dentist.
- Patients who are unable to open their mouth or to swallow, who have significant facial swelling (affecting oral intake or breathing) or who are systemically unwell, should be referred directly to ED.

Patients with a dental problem should be assessed by a qualified dental practitioner and not a medical practitioner. A face-to-face assessment by a medical practitioner would only be warranted if there could potentially be another cause for the patient's symptoms.

Face-to-face

- A study in 2015 in Wales discovered an average general medical practice will see 30–48 patients a year with dental problems, despite patients being aware that there is very little a GP can do in managing dental problems[1].
- It is acceptable to assess and examine the patient and document your findings.

Dental problems

Presentation

- The most common presenting symptom will be pain, and more often than not patients will be able to identify the offending tooth. However, referred pain is common and can often mask the culprit.
- Swelling of the face can be a presenting feature.
- Occasionally bleeding from the gums may occur.
- Patients may also present following a dental procedure, having been unable to access their own dentist.

Assessment

- Again, explain to the patient that you are not a dentist and that you are limited in what you can offer.

- It is acceptable to examine the patient.
- Assess and record vital signs.
- Assess the patient's ability to open their mouth and to swallow.
- Document your findings.

Management[2]

- The GMC has stated: "you should prescribe medicines only if you have adequate knowledge of the patient's health and you are satisfied that they serve the patient's needs"[3].
- Always remember you are responsible for any prescriptions you sign and issue.
- It is reasonable to prescribe pain relief.
- Often a patient may ask for antibiotics for toothache; however, not all causes of toothache are due to infections, and antibiotics will not necessarily make the pain go away.
- ALWAYS: advise the patient to see a dentist as soon as possible; the patient may require X-rays or other investigations. Document this advice.
- REFER: to 111 or the local dental triage service or local emergency dentist if available.
- REFER: to ED or the maxillofacial surgeons if the patient is systemically unwell.
- Indemnity insurers may refuse to provide indemnity cover for treatment of conditions outside your expertise and if you do not have adequate knowledge of the condition or the patient.

The *BMJ* published a clinical review in 2015[4]. It emphasised that dental infection is a common and potentially life-threatening condition and that dental abscesses require surgical treatment. It stated:

- Prompt dental surgery should be arranged rather than prescribing unnecessary antibiotics.
- Antibiotics are inappropriate in the absence of signs of spreading infection or systemic upset.
- Patients presenting with signs of sepsis, facial swelling, trismus (lockjaw) or dysphagia should be reviewed by a dental or maxillofacial surgeon without delay.

Summary for acute dental problems

- Dental problems should be managed by a qualified dentist.
- It is reasonable to assess a patient and document your findings.
- It is appropriate to prescribe pain relief.
- Not all causes of toothache will be due to an infection.

References

1. BMA (updated 2024) *Patients presenting with dental problems*. Available at: www.bma.org.uk/advice-and-support/gp-practices/gp-service-provision/patients-presenting-with-dental-problems

2. MDU (2022) *Treating patients with dental problems: advice for GPs*. Available at: www.themdu.com/guidance-and-advice/guides/treating-patients-with-dental-problems

3. GMC (2021) *Good practice in prescribing and managing medicines and devices*. Available at: www.gmc-uk.org/ethical-guidance/ethical-guidance-for-doctors/prescribing-and-managing-medicines-and-devices

4. Robertson, D.P., Keys, W., Rautemaa-Richardson, R. *et al.* (2015) Management of severe acute dental infections. *BMJ*, **350:** h1300. Available at: https://doi.org/10.1136/bmj.h1300

19

Chapter 19: **Musculoskeletal**

"Take care of your body, it is the only place you have to live."
Jim Rohn

Assessment of patients presenting with acute back pain and musculoskeletal problems

Telephone

- Enquire about precipitating factors such as trauma or a sprain.
- Ascertain the area of the body affected, the severity of the pain and the effect on function.
- A detailed history, including a past medical history of cancer or spinal problems, is essential.
- Enquire about skin rashes.
- In some patients this may be a recurrence, so ask about previous management plans and treatments.
- Ask about red flag features associated with back pain.
- Patients who have features suggesting cauda equina syndrome should be referred directly to ED or the spinal surgeons on call.
- Patients with acute trauma, wounds or limb deformities should be referred directly to an urgent treatment centre or ED.
- Video consultations can be used to assess the skin, deformities and joint movements.

Face-to-face

- Have a low threshold for face-to-face assessments in the elderly and those who present with no obvious cause for their pain.
- Some patients with back pain will have vague symptoms, and signs may be evolving, so consider a face-to-face assessment if this is the case.
- Document positive and negative findings.

Musculoskeletal strains and sprains

Presentation

- The onset will usually be precipitated by activity.
- The patient may be able to recall the exact time the pain occurred and the activity that caused its onset.
- Characteristically the pain will be localised and specific movements will trigger the pain or make it worse.

- Muscular chest wall pain will be worse on deep breathing, coughing, sneezing and on exertion.
- Associated features such as sweating, haemoptysis, dyspnoea and palpitations are absent with chest wall pain, helping to differentiate it from cardiac and pulmonary causes of chest pain.

A face-to-face examination will assist in confirming the diagnosis, although will not always be necessary.

Assessment

- It is important to examine the skin, as shingles affecting the thoracic dermatomes can present with chest pain.
- For chest wall pain cardiovascular and respiratory examination will be normal, including basic observations.
- There may be a localised area of tenderness; characteristically exerting the affected muscle or joint against resistance will exacerbate or trigger the pain.
- X-rays are not required unless bony injury or pathology is suspected.
- If a pneumothorax or haemothorax is suspected with chest wall pain, chest X-rays should be requested.

Management

- The mainstay of soft tissue injuries is rest, ice and analgesia.
- Chest wall injuries can be managed with reassurance, analgesia and deep breathing exercises (for example 5 deep breaths 5 times a day × 5 days).
- Resolution can take 4–6 weeks and if recovery is not complete after this time, the patient should be advised to speak to their own GP.

Costochondritis

Presentation

- This refers to inflammation of the ribcage. The exact aetiology is unknown; however, viral infections have been hypothesised to be the cause.
- The patient will present with pleuritic chest pain, often localised to the costochondral junction.
- Dyspnoea is rare and patients will be well.

Assessment

- Observations will be within normal range.
- Auscultation of the lung fields will be normal.
- There may be tenderness over the affected area.

Management

- Symptoms resolve within 2–3 weeks and regular analgesia is advised.

Rib fractures

Presentation

- There will be a history of significant trauma or a fall.
- Pain will often be severe and will affect the rate and depth of breathing.
- There may be bruising over the affected area.
- The presence of haemoptysis suggests an underlying lung injury.

Assessment

- Rib fractures can be diagnosed clinically; localised tenderness and an audible click (heard with the stethoscope) over the affected area can help clinch the diagnosis.
- Observations will usually be within normal range unless the patient is in severe pain or if lung injury has occurred, in which case tachycardia and tachypnoea may be evident.

Management

- Rib fractures can be extremely painful and opioid analgesia may be required to control the pain.
- The patient should be advised to undertake deep breathing exercises, as poor expansion of the lungs leads to dead spaces of air and can predispose to pneumonia.
- Resolution can take 6–8 weeks.
- X-rays are not required (unless a pneumothorax or haemothorax is suspected) as they do not alter management.

Temporomandibular joint (TMJ) disorder or dysfunction

Presentation

- This refers to pain and dysfunction of the TMJ and muscles of mastication.
- Onset tends to be gradual and it can present with various symptoms including pain around the jaw, neck, temple and ear.
- Opening or closing the mouth may be painful.
- Patients can often present believing they have an ear infection.
- Common predisposers will be chewing gum or hard foods as well as psychological and emotional stress.

Although a detailed history can be taken over the phone and TMJ dysfunction suspected, often a face-to-face assessment will be required – firstly to rule out other causes of pain around the TMJ and also to assess the TMJ itself.

Assessment

- Patients will be well with normal observations.
- There may be clicking or popping, grinding or hissing noises on moving the jaw.
- Palpation of the TMJ on opening and closing the mouth may reveal a clicking sensation.

- Rarely, there may be swelling and tenderness around the TMJ and it may lock on opening the mouth.

Management

- This is based on reassurance, addressing predisposing factors, massage of the joint, and pain relief such as ibuprofen 400mg TDS PC.
- The majority of patients will get better within a few weeks.

Acute back pain

Presentation

- Acute and chronic back pain are common conditions; the estimated lifetime prevalence is 84%, with one-third of the UK population being affected each year[1].
- The lower back is the most common area affected and the paralumbar muscles, ligaments and facet joints are the usual suspects; occasionally it can be from a discogenic cause.
- Key questions to focus on are onset (gradual or sudden), trauma, triggers, alleviating factors and radiation to other parts of the body.
- Essential red flag features to exclude are bowel or bladder problems (notably incontinence and loss of the urge to micturate) and limb weakness.
- The presence of red flag features indicates cauda equina and warrants an immediate referral to hospital.
- Thoracic spine pain is also considered a red flag feature, and if a patient presents with this without an obvious cause, further investigation is warranted.

Assessment[2]

- A thorough examination is important, including general observations.
- Other serious causes should be considered, such as a dissecting aortic aneurysm.
- Inspection of the skin is also vital in order to rule out skin conditions such as shingles or an infection, which may be responsible for the pain.
- The range of movement should be assessed with the patient standing and also sitting down.
- Pain on flexion will indicate a muscular or disc problem, whereas pain on extension indicates a facet joint problem.
- It is important to remember back pain can be multifactorial; it can originate from a combination of structures and an initial insult can trigger a cascade of events. For example, a facet joint sprain can result in inflammation leading to irritation of the nerve roots, often leading to paralumbar spasm.
- Vertebral tenderness is a red flag feature and warrants further investigation.
- Examination of the lower limbs is essential.
- Positive and negative findings should be documented.
- X-rays should be requested if a bony injury is suspected or if there is vertebral tenderness. There should also be a low threshold for requesting X-rays in the elderly, those with a history of or active neoplastic disease, or patients presenting with thoracic spine pain.

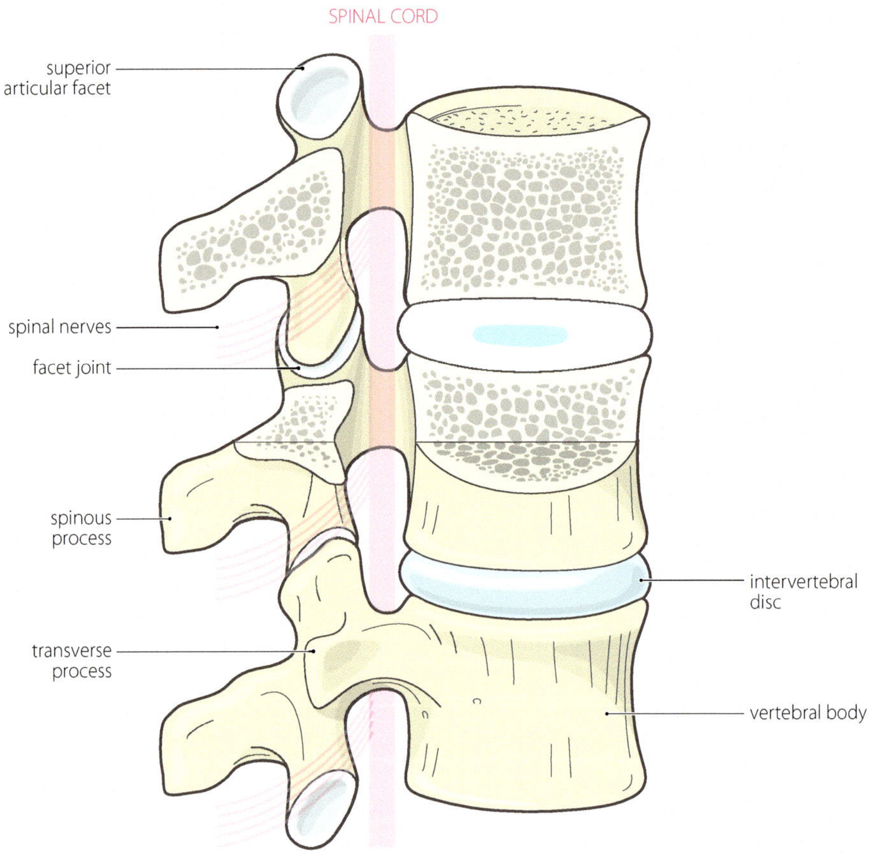

Fig 19.1: The anatomy of the vertebrae.

Reproduced from *Anatomy & Physiology: an introduction for nursing and healthcare* (Minett and Ginesi, 2020), with permission from Lantern Publishing.

Management[2],[3]

- This involves analgesia; common agents are paracetamol, NSAIDs (ibuprofen, naproxen), opiates (codeine) and muscle relaxants (diazepam, baclofen) to alleviate muscle spasm. Neuropathic pain can be managed with a short course of amitriptyline.
- Patients should be advised of sinister features to look out for, such as bowel or bladder disturbances, and advised to follow up with their own GP if symptoms are not better in a few weeks.
- Over time, the underlying or contributory factors such as weak core muscles should be addressed.

Red flag features for back pain

- Age over 50 years
- Thoracic back pain
- Pain occurring at night
- High-impact trauma
- Tenderness over a vertebral body
- Weight loss
- A past or active history of cancer
- Bowel or bladder disturbances
- Limb weakness
- A high temperature

Summary for musculoskeletal

- Patients with limb deformities or wounds should be referred to an urgent treatment centre or ED for assessment.
- Patients presenting with chest wall trauma who are suspected of having a pneumothorax or a haemothorax should have a chest X-ray to rule these out.
- Back pain has a lifetime prevalence of 84%, with one-third of the UK population affected every year. A trigger can result in a domino effect with multiple areas affected, giving rise to different types of pain.
- Patients with back pain should always be assessed for cauda equina syndrome, as a delayed diagnosis can cause irreversible damage[4].
- Pain is not always a feature of cauda equina syndrome; symptoms and signs can evolve with time.
- Positive and negative findings of the assessment should be documented.

References

1. Walker, B.F. (2000) The prevalence of low back pain: a systematic review of the literature from 1966 to 1998. *J Spinal Disord*, **13(3):** 205–217.

2. NICE (updated 2020) *Low back pain and sciatica in over 16s: assessment and management* [NG59]. Available at: www.nice.org.uk/guidance/ng59

3. Macfarlane, G.J., Jones, G.T. and Hannaford, P.C. (2006) Managing low back pain presenting to primary care: where do we go from here? *Pain*, **122(3):** 219–222.

4. MDU (2017) *Why are unscheduled or out of hours consultations more risky?*

20

Chapter 20: **Women's health**

"Whatever women do they must do twice as well as men to be thought half as good. Luckily, this is not difficult."
Charlotte Whitton

Assessment of women presenting with acute gynaecological and obstetric conditions

Telephone

- A detailed history over the phone is essential.
- Enquire about previous gynaecological and obstetric problems, along with any past or current medical problems.
- If the call is regarding an obstetric problem, enquire about any ultrasound scans and investigations in the current pregnancy.
- There is a limited role for video consultations when assessing women with acute gynaecological and obstetric problems.

Face-to-face

- Women in severe pain or with heavy vaginal bleeding will require a face-to-face assessment.
- A general examination is mandatory.
- Always perform a urinalysis and a urine pregnancy test in women who are of childbearing age and present with abdominal or pelvic pain.

Vaginal candidiasis and vulvitis

Presentation and assessment

- Symptoms will be pruritus and a sensation of soreness or burning in and around the introitus. Dysuria may also be present, along with leucocytes on urine dipstick.
- Patients can be misdiagnosed as having a UTI and prescribed antibiotics, often propagating symptoms.
- The possibility of STIs such as herpes simplex should also be considered.
- A face-to-face consultation is rarely required.

Management

- Treatment options for vaginal candidiasis are available over the counter and include clotrimazole cream, clotrimazole pessaries and oral fluconazole tablets.
- Patients may also benefit from an antifungal cream in combination with a topical corticosteroid such as Canesten HC BD × 7 days or Daktacort BD × 7 days.
- Resolution is expected within 10 days; if this does not occur consider a physical examination and low vaginal swabs, especially if there is a vaginal discharge.

Vulvitis is common in young girls and the symptoms can mimic cystitis.

Leucocytes on urine dipstick are also a common finding.

Bartholin's cyst and abscess

Presentation

- Bartholin's glands are a pair of glands that lie on either side of the introitus and are responsible for maintaining the moisture of the vagina.
- The ducts of the glands can occasionally become blocked or inflamed, leading to the formation of Bartholin's cysts.
- Although the cysts can be asymptomatic they can become infected, resulting in pain, swelling and tenderness.
- Infection can also give rise to abscess formation and systemic symptoms.

Women suspected of having infected Bartholin's cysts should be prescribed antibiotics. If symptoms are mild and have resolved with oral antibiotics in the past, then antibiotics can be prescribed over the phone – provided the patient is also systemically well and both the patient and clinician are confident an abscess has not formed. If the above criteria have not been met, a face-to-face assessment is recommended.

Assessment

- Check general observations to ensure there is no systemic infection.
- The gland will be swollen, inflamed and very tender.
- Assess for the presence of an abscess, which will present as a relatively firm, fluctuant, tender and warm swelling around the gland.

Management

- Asymptomatic cysts can be left alone.
- Infected cysts can be treated with flucloxacillin 500mg QDS × 7 days or erythromycin 500mg QDS × 7 days.
- If an abscess has developed or the patient is systemically unwell, a referral to the on-call gynaecology team should be made.

Pelvic inflammatory disease (PID)

Presentation

- PID is rare in women who are sexually inactive, hence enquiring about a sexual history is important.
- Women with PID will have pelvic pain, pyrexia and an offensive vaginal discharge.

Women with PID can be extremely unwell; for this reason a face-to-face assessment is recommended.

Assessment

- The patient may be systemically unwell with tachycardia, a high temperature, diaphoresis and pallor.
- Pelvic tenderness and guarding will be present on examination.
- Vaginal swabs and, if possible, endocervical swabs should be taken and sent for microscopy, culture and sensitivity.

Management[1]

- Pain relief is essential, with a combination of ibuprofen 400mg TDS and co-codamol 30/500mg 2 tablets QDS being an appropriate initial regimen.
- Antibiotics should be commenced in all women with suspected PID.
- First-line antibiotics are ofloxacin 400mg BD in combination with metronidazole 400mg BD × 14 days.
- If there is a high risk of gonorrhoea, a combination of ceftriaxone 500mg IM stat, doxycycline 100mg PO BD and metronidazole 400mg PO BD × 14 days are the antibiotics of choice.
- If the patient is systemically unwell or immunocompromised or unable to take oral medication, a referral to the on-call gynaecologist should be made.

Emergency contraception

Presentation and assessment

- It is important to obtain a detailed history; the patient should be asked about the last menstrual period, the date and time unprotected sexual intercourse took place and whether ejaculation occurred.
- Women with a 28-day cycle will usually ovulate between days 7 and 21 of their cycles.
- Although spermatozoa can survive for 72 hours in the vagina, intercourse outside of days 7 to 21 of the menstrual cycle is unlikely to result in pregnancy.

A physical examination is not required.

Management

- Based on the history, emergency contraception will not always be required.
- If emergency contraception is required the options are: Levonelle (which can be taken orally 72 hours after intercourse; note that the dose may need to be doubled in women who weigh >70kg or have a BMI >26kg/m^2), EllaOne (which can be taken orally 5 days after intercourse) or the IUD (this can be fitted up to 5 days after intercourse).
- The IUD is the most effective form of emergency contraception but requires a trained healthcare professional to fit it.
- Women should be advised that their next period may be early or late and if it is late, to undertake a pregnancy test.

Hyperemesis gravidarum

Presentation

- Nausea and vomiting in pregnancy is common, affecting around 70% of women.
- Hyperemesis gravidarum refers to excessive vomiting in pregnancy and this can affect 1.5% of women.

A face-to-face assessment for women suspected of having hyperemesis gravidarum should be undertaken to assess for the presence and severity of dehydration as well as concomitant conditions such as a UTI, which may be contributing to the excessive vomiting.

Assessment

- A general examination assessing pulse, blood pressure, capillary glucose, temperature, oxygen saturations and respiratory rate is mandatory.
- Assess the mucous membranes.
- Weigh the patient.
- Assess the urine for ketones.

Management [2]

- Nausea and vomiting in pregnancy can be managed in the community with oral rehydration and oral anti-emetics – common agents are cyclizine 50mg TDS, metoclopramide 10mg TDS (be mindful of extrapyramidal side-effects, hence this is considered second-line) and ondansetron 4mg TDS.
- Complementary therapies such as oral ginger, thiamine, acupuncture and hypnotherapy have also been proposed, although efficacy has not been evidenced.
- Failure to respond to oral anti-emetics, dehydration, loss of ≥5% of body weight or the presence of ketones in the urine are all indicators for inpatient management and the patient should be referred to the on-call gynaecology team.
- It is important to look for and manage concomitant and underlying conditions such as gastritis and urinary tract infections.

Criteria for referral to hospital for hyperemesis gravidarum

- No response to oral anti-emetics
- Dehydration (dry mucous membranes, dry tongue, sunken eyes)
- Tachycardia
- Loss of ≥5% of body weight
- Hypoglycaemia
- Ketones in the urine

Ectopic pregnancy

Presentation [3],[4]

- Risk factors for an ectopic pregnancy include a previous ectopic pregnancy, a history of pelvic surgery, and a history of PID or chlamydia.

- Most women will present with features at 6–8 weeks of gestation.
- Typical features are pelvic or abdominal pain, vaginal bleeding and shoulder tip pain.
- It should be noted that an ectopic pregnancy can be asymptomatic; it is only when complications arise that symptoms will manifest themselves.

All women with a suspected ectopic pregnancy will require a face-to-face assessment. If there are features to suggest complications (shoulder tip pain, severe pelvic pain, heavy vaginal bleeding) then an emergency ambulance should be arranged immediately.

Assessment

- A general examination, including assessment of the pulse and blood pressure, is important to rule out excessive blood loss and hypovolaemia due to a ruptured ectopic pregnancy.
- A urine pregnancy test will be positive (but not always!).
- Examination will show pelvic or lower abdominal tenderness and possibly guarding.
- Bimanual examination will reveal cervical excitation and adnexal tenderness.

Management

- All women with a suspected ectopic pregnancy should be referred to the on-call gynaecology team as it is a potentially life-threatening condition.
- An important point to remember is that an ectopic pregnancy can present without all of the above features; on rare occasions the urinary pregnancy test can also be negative, hence if there is a high index of suspicion the patient should always be referred to the on-call gynaecology team for further examination and investigations.

Features of an ectopic pregnancy

- Risk factors – previous ectopic, pelvic surgery, a history of PID
- Pain
- Vaginal bleeding
- Shoulder tip pain
- Lower abdominal tenderness +/– guarding
- Cervical excitation
- Adnexal tenderness
- Positive urinary pregnancy test (not always!)

Threatened miscarriage

Presentation

- The patient may have already had a dating scan which confirms an intrauterine pregnancy, hence eliminating the possibility of an ectopic pregnancy.
- Vaginal bleeding is present, and pain can be variable in intensity and duration.

Not all women will require a face-to-face assessment. If an ectopic pregnancy has been ruled out (normal dating scan showing a viable intrauterine pregnancy) and the pain or bleeding is not excessive, consider a direct referral to the early pregnancy unit.

However, if the pain or bleeding is excessive or there are suspicions regarding an ectopic pregnancy (risk factors such as a previous ectopic pregnancy), a face-to-face assessment is warranted.

Assessment and management[3]

- If the patient's general observations are within normal range and an ectopic pregnancy has been excluded, they can be followed up in the early pregnancy unit at their local hospital.
- This should be booked by the clinician who is assessing the patient and clear instructions should be given to the patient.
- Whilst waiting for the appointment the patient should be advised to rest and if she has any concerns she should seek medical attention via 111 or her own GP.
- It is important family members or friends are nearby.
- If the patient is generally unwell or if the vaginal bleeding is heavy, the patient should be referred to the on-call gynaecology team.
- This will undoubtedly be a stressful and traumatic time for the woman so an empathetic approach is essential.

Acute pelvic pain

All women with acute pelvic pain should be assessed face-to-face, as in some cases the causes can be potentially life-threatening.

- Acute pelvic pain can be due to a number of gynaecological causes; some of these have already been mentioned.
- Other causes include endometriosis, endometritis, ovarian cyst rupture, ovarian cyst haemorrhage, ovarian cyst torsion and ovarian torsion.
- If the patient is systemically unwell or oral analgesia is ineffective, the patient should be referred to the on-call gynaecologist.

Mastitis and breast abscess

Presentation

- This refers to inflammation of the breast tissue.
- It is more common in women who are lactating.
- It can be due to infectious or non-infectious causes; clinically it can be difficult to distinguish between the two.
- Presenting features will be breast pain, redness, swelling, firmness and tenderness.

In an OOH setting lactating mothers may often have already discussed their symptoms with the midwife or health visitor and will often be referred to the OOH primary care services to request antibiotics. Provided the patient is systemically well and the triaging clinician is confident that the complication of a breast abscess is not present, then antibiotics can be prescribed over the phone. If there is any doubt with regard to systemic features or the presence of a breast abscess, a face-to-face assessment should be arranged.

Assessment

- Assess and document general observations.
- Features suggesting an infectious cause are pyrexia, purulent nipple discharge, and failure of symptoms to resolve after expression of breast milk.
- Although not routinely done in primary care, a sample of breast milk can be sent for culture of microorganisms to determine whether the mastitis is infectious and to determine the causative organism.
- A breast abscess will present as a fluctuant, painful and tender lump.

Management

- Advise analgesia and loose-fitting clothing.
- If non-infectious mastitis is suspected, then expressing breast milk in conjunction with conservative measures mentioned above can alleviate symptoms.
- If infectious mastitis is suspected, prescribe antibiotics: flucloxacillin 500mg QDS × 14 days or clarithromycin 500mg BD × 14 days in those who are allergic to penicillin.
- Flucloxacillin is appropriate to use in breastfeeding mothers; clarithromycin will be present in breast milk and should only be used if the benefits outweigh this risk.
- For non-lactating women, prescribe co-amoxiclav 500/125mg TDS × 10–14 days or clarithromycin 500mg BD and metronidazole 400mg TDS × 10–14 days in those who are allergic to penicillin.
- Women who are systemically unwell or have a breast abscess should be referred to the on-call breast or general surgeons.

Summary for women's health

- Vulvitis can mimic symptoms of a UTI and vice versa.
- 1.5% of pregnant women will suffer from hyperemesis gravidarum.
- Women who have an ectopic pregnancy can have a negative urinary pregnancy test.
- Women with severe and acute pelvic pain of unknown aetiology, or whose pain is uncontrolled with oral pain relief, should be referred to hospital.

References

1. NICE (revised 2024) *Pelvic inflammatory disease* – Management. Available at: https://cks.nice.org.uk/pelvic-inflammatory-disease#!scenario

2. Royal College of Obstetricians & Gynaecologists (2016) *The management of nausea and vomiting of pregnancy and hyperemesis gravidarum* (GTG No. 69). Available at: www.rcog.org.uk/en/guidelines-research-services/guidelines/gtg69/

3. Royal College of Obstetricians & Gynaecologists (2016) *Diagnosis and management of ectopic pregnancy* (GTG No. 21). Available at: www.rcog.org.uk/en/guidelines-research-services/guidelines/gtg21/

4. NICE (2012) *Ectopic pregnancy and miscarriage: diagnosis and initial management* [CG154]. Available at: www.nice.org.uk/guidance/cg154

Chapter 21: **Men's health**

"Nearly all men can stand adversity, but if you want to test a man's character, give him power."
Abraham Lincoln

Assessment of acute male genital conditions

Telephone

- A detailed history can be taken over the phone.
- Enquire about systemic symptoms such as pyrexia, which indicates an infection.
- Enquire about previous episodes, as certain conditions such as acute prostatitis can be recurrent.
- With regard to testicular pain, the patient's age will aid in determining the diagnosis. Testicular torsion is more common in boys and adolescents and orchitis is more common in older sexually active men.
- Video consultations will be of limited use.
- Have a low threshold for face-to-face assessments.

Face-to-face

A face-to-face assessment would be required in the following situations:

- The diagnosis is unclear.
- The presence of systemic features such as a high temperature, and the need to assess for markers of sepsis.
- There are suspected complications such as acute urinary retention.

Testicular torsion

Presentation

- This refers to twisting of the testis.
- Testicular torsion is more common amongst young men and boys.
- It can cause cessation of the blood supply to the testis and the consequence is testicular infarction.
- Those affected will complain of intense pain around the affected testis.
- Onset of symptoms is acute and there may be a history of trauma or physical exertion, such as cycling or running.

Patients with suspected testicular torsion should have a face-to-face assessment.

Assessment[1]

- On examination the affected testis will be tense, tender and high up in the scrotum.
- Testicular infarction and atrophy can occur if testicular torsion is left untreated for more than 6 hours.

Management

- Patients should be referred to the on-call general surgical team or urology team for immediate assessment.

Orchitis and epididymitis

Presentation

- Orchitis refers to infection of the testis, and epididymitis refers to infection of the epididymis.
- Often the two conditions manifest together.
- Patients will usually be young or middle-aged men who are sexually active, although there will always be exceptions.
- Those affected may report a high temperature and an insidious onset of pain and feeling generally unwell, thus differentiating it from testicular torsion.

Although orchitis and epididymitis can be suspected over the phone, a face-to-face assessment is recommended. This will allow an assessment of general observations as well as assessing and ruling out the possibility of testicular torsion.

Assessment

- On examination the testis or epididymis will feel warm and be exquisitely tender; however, it will remain free and mobile within the scrotum, thereby helping to differentiate it from testicular torsion.
- The patient may have mild pyrexia and associated tachycardia.

Management[2]

- Although some cases can be viral and self-limiting, oral antibiotics are recommended.
- Commonly prescribed antibiotics are ofloxacin 200mg BD × 14 days, or doxycycline 100mg BD × 14 days.
- If gonorrhoea or chlamydia is suspected to be the cause, the patient should be referred to the sexual health clinic.

Differences between testicular torsion and orchitis

Testicular torsion	vs.	*Orchitis*
Boys and adolescents		Young and middle-aged men
History of trauma or exertion		Sexually active
Sudden onset		Gradual onset
Severe pain		Dull ache
Normal temperature		Low-grade pyrexia
Tense and tender testis		Tender testis +/– epididymis
Immobile testis		Mobile testis
Refer to hospital		Antibiotics and analgesia

Red flags in men presenting with a testicular swelling

All male patients with a testicular swelling of more than 2 weeks' duration and with no obvious cause should be referred for an ultrasound scan to rule out testicular tumours.

Balanitis and posthitis

Presentation

- Balanitis refers to inflammation of the glans (head of the penis) and posthitis refers to inflammation of the foreskin. The two conditions often coexist.
- It is more common in young men and boys.
- A tight foreskin can often be a precipitating factor.
- Balanitis is usually caused by local irritation or an infection, commonly candidal or bacterial – the latter often presenting with a purulent discharge.

In most cases the diagnosis can be made over the phone; a video consultation may also help.

A face-to-face assessment would be required if there are concerns of a concomitant UTI or if the person is unable to pass urine.

Assessment

- The patient will usually be systemically well.
- The foreskin will be swollen and inflamed.
- It is important to ensure the patient can pass urine freely, as failure to do so would be an indication for referral to hospital.

Management

- Mild candidal balanitis can be managed with a topical antifungal and steroid cream such as Daktacort applied 3 times a day × 7 days or Canesten HC applied 3 times a day × 7 days.
- Oral fluconazole 150mg as a one-off dose may also help eradicate the fungal infection.
- Bacterial infections (suggested by the presence of a purulent and/or offensive discharge) should be managed with oral antibiotics such as flucloxacillin 500mg QDS × 7 days or a macrolide antibiotic such as clarithromycin 500mg BD × 7 days in those who are allergic to penicillin.
- Metronidazole 400mg TDS × 7 days may be required if *Gardnerella* balanitis is suspected (a characteristic fishy odour is present in the discharge).

Urethritis

Presentation

- Men who have urethritis may present suspecting they have a urine infection.
- However, discerning features are penile pain, dysuria and a urethral discharge.
- It is more common in men who have unprotected intercourse.

Often the symptoms will mimic those of a lower UTI; in such cases a face-to-face assessment will be required, primarily to examine the urethral meatus and also to perform a urinalysis.

Assessment

- On examination the urethral meatus will appear inflamed and there will be a discharge.
- There may also be inguinal lymphadenopathy.
- Urine dipstick may reveal the presence of leucocytes in the urine (often from contamination as urine passes through the urethra).
- The patient will be systemically well.

Management[3]

- Ideally all men who present with urethritis should be referred for a sexual health screen; however, in an OOH setting this may not be possible and often patients will prefer to have treatment as soon as possible.
- In such cases doxycycline 100mg BD × 7 days can be prescribed; however, the patient should be advised to follow up with his own GP and consider attending a sexual health clinic.

Urethritis symptoms can mimic those of a UTI; hence it is important to examine the penis and urethral meatus in men who present with dysuria.

Acute prostatitis

Presentation[4]

- Acute prostatitis refers to inflammation (not always due to infection) of the prostate gland.
- This is a small walnut-sized gland found beneath the bladder in men.
- Although prostate cancer and benign prostate hypertrophy are conditions associated with older men, prostatitis is more common amongst men aged between 30 and 50 years.
- It can be asymptomatic; however, acute bacterial prostatitis will usually present with pelvic, perineal or lower abdominal pain.
- Pyrexia may be present, and some men may notice haematospermia (blood in the semen).
- It may also present with dysuria, frequency of micturition and occasionally acute urinary retention.

Often the diagnosis is one of exclusion and it is important to rule out other causes of abdominal or pelvic pain, such as a UTI.

A face-to-face assessment should be undertaken to rule out other causes of symptoms and to assess for potential complications.

Assessment[4],[5]

- General examination is important to rule out features of sepsis or acute urinary retention.
- Patients who present with these features should be referred to the on-call urology team or ED.
- A rectal examination may reveal an enlarged and tender prostate gland.

Management[5]

- Mild to moderate cases of infective acute prostatitis can be managed in the community with oral antibiotics; the antibiotics of choice are ciprofloxacin 500mg BD or trimethoprim 200mg BD × 14 days.
- Hydration and analgesia should be advised.
- Symptoms can take several weeks to settle, and patients should be advised of this.
- Oral NSAIDs will help with pain and assist in reducing inflammation.
- Advise the patient that if during the recovery period there are any features to suggest complications or if he has any concerns, he should seek medical attention immediately.

Summary for men's health

- Testicular infarction can occur if testicular torsion is left untreated for more than 6 hours.
- Testicular pain with a free and mobile testis in the scrotum is likely to be due to orchitis, as opposed to testicular torsion.
- Urethritis may be mistaken for a urinary tract infection.
- Acute prostatitis can be a cause of perineal pain in men aged 30 to 50 years.

References

1. NICE (revised 2024) *Scrotal pain and swelling*. Available at: https://cks.nice.org.uk/scrotal-pain-and-swelling

2. Nicholson, A., Rait, G., Murray-Thomas, T. *et al.* (2010) Management of epididymo-orchitis in primary care: results from a large UK primary care database. *Br J Gen Pract*, **60(579):** e407–e422.

3. NICE (revised 2024) *Urethritis – male*. Available at: https://cks.nice.org.uk/urethritis-male#!scenario

4. Cooper, A. and Rees, J. (2014) New guideline will aid GPs in diagnosis and treatment of prostatitis. *Guidelines in Practice*, **17(12):** 9–20.

5. NICE (revised 2024) *Prostatitis – acute* – Management. Available at: https://cks.nice.org.uk/prostatitis-acute#!scenario

22

Chapter 22: **Paediatrics**

"Too many people grow up. That's the real trouble with the world, too many people grow up. They forget. They don't remember what it's like to be 12 years old. They patronize, they treat children as inferiors. Well I won't do that."

Walt Disney

Assessment of children

Important notes

- Children can become unwell very quickly and often will not be able to articulate their symptoms. Although recovery can be just as quick, extra care should be taken when assessing them.
- Safety-netting is extremely important and it is helpful to explain specific features or complications parents should look out for, an example being drowsiness post headaches.
- My advice to parents has always been "if you have any concerns you must call back".
- Written advice in the form of patient leaflets and booklets can also help.
- Any verbal or written advice given to parents should be documented in the patient's medical notes.

Telephone

- A detailed history of the presenting complaint is essential, along with any associated symptoms and potential red flag features such as a non-blanching rash.
- Older children may be able to provide a history themselves, therefore take the opportunity to speak to the child.
- Access any summary care records and previous encounters; also determine if the child is on the child protection register.
- It helps to query whether the child is feeding well and to quantify the amount of oral intake. Producing urine and wet nappies are reassuring signs.
- Ask about noisy breathing, colour and also general behaviour.
- Deviation from normal behaviour indicates the child is not well.
- Some parents will be able to undertake a basic assessment and will be able to assess for red flag features such as a non-blanching rash, recessions or nasal flaring.
- Some parents may have appropriate equipment to check basic observations such as temperature, pulse rate, respiratory rate and oxygen saturations (adult pulse oximeters will not give an accurate reading in children).
- If there are alarming features such as an increased respiratory rate, intercostal recessions or a very high temperature (red flag features), consider a direct referral to hospital via ambulance.

- Occasionally you may be able to hear the child in the background; document this and whether the child sounds well or is in pain.
- It also helps to ask parents what they are concerned about and whether there are specific features they find alarming.
- Ask about previous episodes of the illness and how they were managed.
- Ask parents what the child is doing whilst you are on the phone to them.
- Video consultations will allow you to obtain a general impression as to whether the child is well or unwell.
- Have an extremely low threshold for face-to-face assessments in children.
- Tactfully enquire about any safeguarding issues or if the child is known to social services. If the answer is yes, consider a face-to-face appointment to explore the presenting symptoms and history further.

Face-to-face

- A head-to-toe assessment is recommended.
- Always document your subjective assessment findings, e.g. alert, well, bouncing off walls, playful, running, etc.
- Always assess and document objective findings such as temperature, pulse, blood pressure (if possible), SpO_2 (if possible), central capillary refill time (this should be <2 seconds), and respiratory rate.
- Is there a rash? Is it blanching?
- Assess the anterior fontanelle: a sunken fontanelle is a sign of dehydration; a bulging fontanelle is a sign of raised intracranial pressure.
- Consider checking capillary glucose levels for certain conditions; for example, gastroenteritis can cause hypoglycaemia even in well-hydrated children.
- Ask yourself whether abdominal pain could be due to diabetic ketoacidosis.
- Bear in mind children can become unwell very quickly.
- Have a very low threshold for referral to the on-call paediatricians.
- If the child has had three or more contacts with healthcare professionals for the same acute problem, consider referral to the on-call paediatricians.
- As parental anxiety plays a large role in developing and implementing a management plan, it is important to assess whether the parents feel comfortable with taking their child home.

Become familiar with normal paediatric vital signs

Age group	Heart rate (bpm)	Respirations/min	Systolic BP (mmHg)
Preterm	120–180	50–70	40–60
Newborn (0 to 1 month)	100–160	35–55	50–70
Infant (1 to 12 months)	80–140	30–40	70–100
Toddler (1 to 3 years)	80–130	20–30	70–110
Preschool (3 to 6 years)	80–110	20–30	80–110
School age (6 to 12 years)	70–100	18–24	80–120
Adolescents (12+ years)	60–90	14–22	100–120

Adapted with permission from *Nelson Textbook of Pediatrics*, 18th edition Kliegman, R.M. (ed.), © Saunders Elsevier (2007).

Children presenting with a high temperature

Presentation[1],[2]

- Ask parents if they have measured the temperature with a thermometer, and what part of the body the temperature has been taken from.
- A true high temperature will be associated with tachycardia.
- As a rule of thumb a 1°C rise in core temperature will result in an increase in the resting heart rate of 10 beats per minute.
- Obtaining a system-specific history may assist in identifying the source of the high temperature.
- Enquire about any measures the parents have taken to control the temperature.
- Ask about red flag features, such as a non-blanching rash, or features suggestive of sepsis, such as a temperature >40°C.
- If red flag features are present, consider a direct referral to hospital via ambulance.
- Viral infections are the most common cause of a high temperature in children.
- Most children with mild pyrexia for <72 hours can be managed with regular paracetamol, ibuprofen and cool fluids taken orally.

Have a low threshold for assessing children face-to-face, especially if you are unable to obtain a clear history, or if you are unable to determine the cause of the high temperature, or you are unable to determine how unwell the child is over the phone.

Assessment

- Examine the child head to toe after removing their clothing.
- Assess vital signs.
- Areas to assess are: fontanelles, mucous membranes, sclera, ears (including tympanic membranes), pharynx, tonsils, cervical glands, cardiovascular examination, capillary refill time, respiratory examination, abdominal examination, genitalia, hips, feet and hands, skin, and midstream urine sample for urinalysis.

Management

- Pyrexia of unknown origin in a child requires a referral to the on-call paediatricians.
- If a source has been identified, this should be treated.
- Viral infections will be self-limiting and parents can be reassured and given advice with regard to managing the high temperature and ensuring hydration.
- A tight safety-net should be applied with clear instructions on timeframes and when you expect the child to be better.
- An example statement could be "if your son/daughter is not better in 48 hours, or if they become worse, or if you have any concerns whatsoever, you must return or call us via telephone".
- Once a cause has been identified and treatment commenced, the high temperature can be managed with paracetamol and ibuprofen in combination.
- Cool fluids taken orally, ice lollies, fans and ensuring the child wears loose clothing and as few layers as possible will also help.

Red flag for children presenting with a high temperature

Children with pyrexia of unknown origin should be referred to hospital.

Croup

Presentation[3],[4]

- Croup is a viral infection of the upper airways, i.e. the larynx and trachea.
- Highest incidence is during autumn to winter and it usually affects children aged 6 months to 3 years of age. However, it can occur outside these age groups and can also affect adults.
- Children will often present with a high temperature and a runny nose.
- Characteristically croup causes a harsh barking cough and occasionally an inspiratory stridor.
- Parents will complain they haven't slept all night and this will be evident on their faces.

Mild cases of croup can be managed with supportive measures such as regular oral fluids, having the child sit upright, anti-pyretic agents and reassurance, which can be given over the phone.

A video consultation may help relieve any parental anxiety and also help the clinician identify any features suggestive of respiratory distress.

Consider a face-to-face assessment if the history is prolonged or there are suspicions the child may be systemically unwell with decreased oral intake.

Assessment

The majority of children will be well on examination.

Although the **modified Westley clinical scoring system** for croup is used primarily for research, it can assist in determining the severity.

Inspiratory stridor	Not present – 0 points	When agitated/active – 1 point	At rest – 2 points
Intercostal recession	Mild – 1 point	Moderate – 2 points	Severe – 3 points
Decreased air entry	None – 0 points	Mildly – 1 point	Severely – 2 points
Cyanosis	None – 0 points	With activity – 4 points	Resting – 5 points
Level of consciousness	Normal – 0 points	Altered – 5 points	
Total score 0–17: • <4 = mild croup • 4–6 = moderate croup • >6 = severe croup			

Management[4]

- For management of mild croup all that is required is reassurance and empathy for fatigued parents. Sitting the child upright and encouraging cool fluids will help.
- Anti-pyretics and analgesia such as paracetamol and ibuprofen will also help relieve any associated symptoms, such as a pyrexia or sore throat.
- Consider oral corticosteroids if croup is causing the child and parents distress or if the symptoms have an unusually prolonged course.
- A delayed prescription for oral corticosteroids can also help allay parental anxieties; advise parents to commence medication if their child is not better in 48 hours.
- Commonly prescribed corticosteroids are prednisolone 1–2mg/kg and dexamethasone 150mcg/kg.
- A stat dose of one of these can be given after assessment; a second dose after 24 hours should be considered if symptoms are persisting.
- Moderate to severe cases, especially if there are signs of respiratory distress (respiratory rate >60, SpO_2 <92% on air) or if there is a risk of dehydration, should be referred to the on-call paediatricians after a stat dose of oral corticosteroids has been given.

Features of severe croup

- Inspiratory stridor
- Decreased air entry
- Cyanosis
- Decreased consciousness
- Respiratory distress

Red flag features (indicating respiratory distress)

- Nasal flaring
- Cyanosis
- Intercostal and subcostal recessions
- Respiratory rate >60 breaths/min
- SpO_2 <92% on air

Bronchiolitis and viral-induced wheeze

Presentation[5]

- Bronchiolitis by definition alludes to inflammation of bronchioles. Bronchiolitis and viral-induced wheeze can manifest simultaneously or present on their own.
- The most common cause is a viral infection, with the main culprit being respiratory syncytial virus (RSV) in 75% of cases.
- Peak incidence is during winter months, with children under 2 years old affected the most.
- Typical features tend to be a high temperature, coryzal symptoms, a cough and a wheeze.
- Symptoms tend to peak between days 3 and 5.

- Enquire about any features of respiratory distress, reduced oral intake and reduced urine output, as these features would indicate moderate to severe bronchiolitis.

Mild cases can be assessed and managed over the phone; however, if there is high parental anxiety, a protracted course or the child is suspected of being unwell, a face-to-face assessment should be arranged.

Assessment

- Assess general observations.
- Assess hydration status.
- Look for signs of respiratory distress; document these and also any negative findings.
- Auscultation of the chest will reveal wheezes and crepitations over the affected lung areas.

Management [4],[5]

- Mild cases will resolve with conservative measures, including anti-pyretics to control a high temperature and fluids to ensure the child remains well hydrated.
- A salbutamol inhaler with a volumatic or aerochamber device can be prescribed; 2 puffs given four times a day × 5 days can help alleviate the wheeze whilst the viral infection abates.
- Indications for referral to the on-call paediatricians include signs of respiratory distress (respiratory rate >60, SpO_2 <92% on air), <50% of normal fluid intake or signs of dehydration, parental concerns, or if the child looks unwell or is at risk of becoming acutely unwell.
- Transfers should be via a category 1 or 2 ambulance and oxygen should be readily available, if not already being administered.
- Unwell children with a wheeze should also be given a salbutamol nebuliser or 10 puffs of a salbutamol inhaler with a spacer whilst waiting for an ambulance to arrive.

Red flag features of bronchiolitis

The presence of these warrants a referral to hospital:

- Respiratory distress
- <50% of normal fluid intake
- Signs of dehydration
- Generally unwell child
- Parental concerns
- Child is at risk of becoming acutely unwell

Gastroenteritis

Presentation

- Commonly this is due to a self-limiting and benign viral infection.
- In children the most common cause is rotavirus (hence the UK's rotavirus immunisation programme). In adults the most common cause is norovirus.

- Although self-limiting and benign, the symptoms of diarrhoea and vomiting can last for several days.
- Enquire about the number of episodes of diarrhoea and vomiting over a specific period of time.
- Ask about when the last episode of each occurred.
- Enquire about pain or red flag features such as blood in the stool.
- Ask parents if the tongue appears dry or moist, or if the fontanelle is sunken.
- Enquire about oral intake and urine output.
- Some parents may be able to give an impression on the hydration status of the child.

A detailed and thorough history over the phone can assist in ascertaining the severity of symptoms as well as the hydration status of the child. A video consultation will also assist in doing this.

Children with mild symptoms who are well hydrated can be managed with telephone advice.

If there are concerns with regard to the hydration status of the child or there are red flag features such as a sunken fontanelle, arrange a face-to-face assessment.

Assessment

- It is essential to identify signs of dehydration, which include a sunken fontanelle, sunken eyes, dry mucous membranes, dry nappies, tachycardia, hypotension and lethargy.
- In children who are listless or appear generally unwell it is important to check the blood glucose levels, as hypoglycaemia is a complication.

Management

- This involves oral rehydration.
    - a fluid challenge can be conducted in the clinic
    - the aim is to encourage 1ml/1kg of electrolyte balanced fluids per hour
    - parents can keep a record of how much fluid has been given; if after 4 hours the child has managed to keep fluids down and the parents are comfortable with taking the child home, the child can be discharged with the advice that if the parents have any concerns, they should return
    - oral rehydration salts such as Dioralyte are available over the counter and should be encouraged, along with sugary fluids and a light diet.
- Use of oral loperamide should be avoided in children.
- If there are any signs of dehydration or if there is dysentery, the child should be referred to the on-call paediatricians.

Features of dehydration in children

- Lethargy
- Sunken fontanelle
- Sunken eyes
- Dry mucous membranes
- Dry nappies
- Tachycardia
- Hypotension

Sepsis

Presentation and assessment[6],[7],[8]

- Sepsis affects 25 000 children in the UK per year.
- Sepsis kills, and it kills very quickly.
- I can recall a child who had been discharged from an ED in the morning, only to be re-admitted less than 12 hours later with sepsis requiring intensive care intervention.
- Predisposers to sepsis include being very young or very old, chronic illnesses such as diabetes mellitus and immunodeficiency.
- Patients who fall within these groups and present with an infection are at increased risk of developing sepsis, and this must be taken into account when assessing and managing these patients.
- Key features include a very high (>39°C) or low temperature (<36°C), rapid shallow breathing or laboured and slow breathing, cyanosis, mottled skin and cold peripheries.
- There may also be features to suggest an underlying cause, such as a bulging fontanelle associated with meningitis or a non-blanching rash associated with meningococcal septicaemia.
- Other features include poor feeding, confusion, listlessness, absent or severely diminished postural tone, tachycardia and hypotension.

Many of the above features can be ascertained over the phone; a video consultation will help but is not necessary – patients with suspected sepsis should be referred to hospital via emergency ambulance.

Management[8]

- Immediate referral to hospital via a category 1 or 2 ambulance should be done without delay.
- If you are with the patient, consider giving IM or IV antibiotics if available and whilst waiting for an ambulance.

Features of sepsis in children[7]

- A very high temperature (>39°C)
- A very low temperature (<36°C)
- Rapid shallow or slow laboured breathing
- Cyanosis
- Mottled skin
- Cold peripheries
- Poor feeding
- Confusion
- Lethargy or listlessness
- Severely diminished postural tone
- Tachycardia
- Hypotension
- Low oxygen saturations
- Also look for underlying causes, e.g. bulging fontanelle

Invasive Group A *Streptococcus* infections

Group A *Streptococcus* (*S. pyogenes*) are bacteria which are spread via respiratory droplets and via direct contact with infected individuals and inanimate objects. They can cause a wide range of infections including erysipelas, pharyngitis, tonsillitis, cellulitis, pneumonia and scarlet fever [9].

Presentation

- Presentation of streptococcal infections depends very much on which parts of the body are infected and to what extent. Common presenting features will be flu-like symptoms such as a sore throat, a high temperature, generalised myalgia, nausea and vomiting [10].
- Scarlet fever will present with a sore throat, high temperature and a generalised rash (erythematous, blanching and with a sandpaper-like texture) and a strawberry tongue (erythematous, swollen with a white exudate).
- A serious sequelae of Group A *Streptococcus* (GAS) infections are invasive Group A *Streptococcus* (iGAS) infections. These occur when there is widespread infection with GAS in normally sterile body sites resulting in bacteraemia and, in rare cases, death. It can also cause necrotising fasciitis, necrotising pneumonia and streptococcal toxic shock syndrome, all of which can be fatal.
- An increased incidence of iGAS infections, especially in children under the age of 10 years was initially noted in the UK in late 2022 [11].
- Both iGAS and scarlet fever are notifiable diseases.

Patients with mild and localised infections such as impetigo can be managed over the phone with the aid of photographs or videos.

Patients who have systemic features such as pyrexia, a rash and generalised malaise, as well as those at high risk of complications (e.g. the young and the elderly) should be offered a face-to-face consultation to determine the type and severity of infection.

Assessment

- Always bear in mind that GAS can cause a wide range of infections, and have the propensity to progress and result in serious illness.
- All patients who are systemically unwell should have their observations taken.
- The presence or absence of a rash should be noted; if a rash is present document the characteristics.

Management [12],[13]

The majority of people with a GAS infection will generally be well and will recover without sequelae.

- Although antigen testing should be obtained prior to prescribing antibiotics, this may not always be possible:
  - In patients who are generally unwell or at risk of becoming seriously unwell (children, elderly, immunocompromised) antibiotics should not be withheld.

  - In those who have a CENTOR score of 3 or 4 (FeverPAIN score of ≥3), antibiotics should be prescribed.
- First line is phenoxymethylpenicillin 500mg qds; in those allergic to penicillin, clarithromycin 500mg bd or erythromicin 500mg qds can be prescribed.
  - For those with a sore throat, a 5 day course of antibiotics is recommended.
  - For those who have scarlet fever or tonsillitis a 10-day course of antibiotics is recommended.
- Supportive measures such as adequate fluid intake, pain relief, anaesthetic lozenges and throat sprays should be advocated.
- Hospital admission is indicated for patients with iGAS and any complications of streptococcal infections such as quinsy, rheumatic fever, necrotising pneumonia and sepsis.
- Patients who present with a suspected GAS infection and who are on immunosuppressant medication should have an urgent FBC arranged. They should also be discussed with the medical team on call; consider commencing antibiotics whilst awaiting results.
- Prophylaxis treatment of close contacts of patients who have proven iGAS should be discussed with local health protection teams.

Summary for paediatrics

- Children can become unwell very quickly, and can recover just as quickly.
- Always complete a head-to-toe examination when assessing an unwell child.
- Consider checking blood glucose levels in unwell children.
- Sepsis affects 25 000 children per year in the UK.
- Consider observing the child for a period of time if possible, or arranging a follow-up call after discharge.
- Make sure parents are comfortable with your management plan and understand who they can contact if they have any concerns.
- Have a low threshold for prescribing antibiotics in vulnerable children who have a GAS infection.
- If an iGAS infection is suspected start antibiotics and refer to hospital urgently.
- Have a low threshold for referring children to hospital.
- If a child is referred to hospital, transport should be via a category 1 or 2 ambulance unless this would cause further delay.

References

1. NICE (updated 2021) *Fever in under 5s: assessment and initial management* [NG143). Available at: www.nice.org.uk/guidance/ng143

2. NICE (revised 2023) *Feverish children – risk assessment and management*. Available at: https://cks.nice.org.uk/topics/feverish-children-risk-assessment-management

3. NICE (revised 2022) *Croup*. Available at: https://cks.nice.org.uk/croup#!background

4. Everard, M.L. (2009) Acute bronchiolitis and croup. *Pediatr. Clin. North Am.* **56(1):** 119–33.

5. NICE (2021) *Bronchiolitis in children: diagnosis and management* [NG9]. Available at: www.nice.org.uk/guidance/ng9

6. NHS (no date) *Sepsis*. Available at: www.nhs.uk/conditions/sepsis/

7. NICE (updated 2024) *Suspected sepsis: recognition, diagnosis and early management* [NG51]. Available at: www.nice.org.uk/guidance/ng51

8. NICE (revised 2024) *Sepsis* – Management. Available at: https://cks.nice.org.uk/sepsis#!scenario

9. UK Health Security Agency (updated 2023) *Group A streptococcus*. Available at: www.gov.uk/government/collections/group-a-streptococcal-infections-guidance-and-data

10. NHS (no date) *Strep A*. Available at: www.nhs.uk/conditions/strep-a/#:~:text=Most%20strep%20A%20infections%20can,infection%20spreading%20to%20other%20people

11. UK Health Security Agency (2023) *Group A streptococcal infections: first update on seasonal activity in England, 2022 to 2023*. Available at: www.gov.uk/government/publications/group-a-streptococcal-infections-activity-during-the-2022-to-2023-season/group-a-streptococcal-infections-first-update-on-seasonal-activity-in-england-2022-to-2023

12. NICE (revised 2024) *Sore throat: acute, management*. Available at: https://cks.nice.org.uk/topics/sore-throat-acute/management/management/

13. NHS (2023) *Group A Streptococcus: reinstatement of NICE sore throat guidance for children and young people and withdrawal of NHS England interim guidance.* Available at: www.england.nhs.uk/wp-content/uploads/2022/12/PRN00247_Group-A-Streptococcus-reinstatement-of-NICE-sore-throat-guidance-for-children-and-young-people-and-wi.pdf

Chapter 23: **Cancer / palliative care**

"We cannot change the outcome but we can affect the journey."
Ann Richardson

During my first few years as a GP, I was surprised at the number of palliative care patients managed in primary care. However, as the years have progressed I have come to realise this is perhaps one of the most important and rewarding aspects of being a primary care clinician and doctor in family medicine. Taking your last breaths on a hospital trolley in a noisy corridor is not the right way to depart this life, and regardless of how you have lived your life, death should be a peaceful and dignified process.

In the UK the community palliative care nurses, Macmillan nurses, hospice at home nurses and district nurses play an invaluable role and should always be involved when caring for patients who are at the end of their life.

It is always good practice to pre-empt end of life care and ensure resources and medication are in place. Failure to do this is really inexcusable. The aim should be to minimise distress to the patient and family. Ideally a discussion regarding resuscitation and escalation of care should have been made by the patient's usual GP. An advance directive or care plan may also be available and can be referred to by emergency healthcare professionals when ascertaining the patient's and family's wishes for end of life care.

Local hospice services will also be available to provide advice and guidance. Consider admission to a hospice if symptoms cannot be managed at home. Always take into account loved ones and family, as they are undoubtedly going through a lot of pain and heartache.

Assessment of patients who are for palliative care[1],[2],[3]

Telephone

- Take a detailed history from the patient; if this is not possible speak to their next of kin.
- Enquire about what symptoms are causing distress.
- Take a detailed medication history.
- Ask about what has already been taken and what is available to the patient and family.
- Ask if palliative care medication is with the patient and whether a district nurse authorisation chart has been signed.
- Ask what support the family have had and whether palliative care nurses are involved.

- Enquire about advance care plans and if there is one in place, ascertain what the wishes of the patient and family are.
- Do not assume there is a 'Do Not Attempt Cardiopulmonary Resuscitation' request in place.
- This will be an extremely distressing time for the patient and family; express empathy.

Provided appropriate medication is in place with an authorisation chart and the district or palliative care nurses are involved, patients can be managed with telephone advice and remote prescribing of appropriate medication.

However, if this is not possible have a very low threshold for a face-to-face assessment, and often but not always a home visit may be required.

Pain management

Assessment and management

- The aim is to start with 'simple' oral analgesia.
- Paracetamol 1g every 6 hours is a good starting point, but may not be enough to control pain for long.
- NSAIDs such as ibuprofen, naproxen and diclofenac can also be used, provided there are no contraindications. Consider prescribing these with a PPI to reduce the risk of adverse GI effects.
- Consider topical analgesia in the form of gels and creams. These are available over the counter and studies have shown very little difference in efficacy between the various types and brands available.
- Should the above measures fail, oral opioid analgesia can be introduced; examples are [4]:
  - codeine 15–60mg every 6 hours
  - co-codamol 8/500 or 30/500 – one or two tablets every 6 hours
  - co-dydramol – one or two tablets every 6 hours
  - oramorph 10mg/5ml – 5ml as required
  - tramadol (CD) 50mg – one or two capsules every 8 hours.
- Co-codamol is a combination of codeine phosphate and paracetamol; co-dydramol is a combination of dihydrocodeine and paracetamol.
- Avoid prescribing a combination of different opiates together, as this increases the risk of respiratory depression.
- For breakthrough pain relief prescribe one-sixth of the total 24-hour dose of opiates. For example, if a patient is taking 36mg of morphine sulphate orally over 24 hours, then the dose for breakthrough pain relief would be 6mg of morphine sulphate.
- Patients can take breakthrough pain relief as often as required, as the aim is to ensure the patient remains as pain-free as possible.
- Analgesia should be titrated upwards until patients no longer require breakthrough pain relief; this is done by calculating the total amount of analgesia (regular + breakthrough) required over a 24-hour period.

- It should be noted that as the regular analgesia dose is titrated upwards, so should the dose of breakthrough analgesia.
- For patients struggling with oral analgesia consider patches, but bear in mind pain will not be controlled instantly, and it will take time for the drug to reach a steady state concentration *in situ*.
- Consider oral adjuncts to opioid analgesia; these may be more effective in managing neuropathic pain. Examples are:
  - amitriptyline, starting at 10mg at night and titrating upwards
  - pregabalin, 50mg three times a day and titrating upwards
  - gabapentin, 300mg once a day and titrating upwards.
- Diazepam (2–5mg every 8 hours) can also be used to treat muscle spasm and anxiety.

The table below indicates the equivalent doses of opioid analgesics.

Analgesic / route	**Dose**
Codeine: PO	100mg
Diamorphine: IM, IV, SC	3mg
Dihydrocodeine: PO	100mg
Hydromorphone: PO	2mg
Morphine: PO	10mg
Morphine: IM, IV, SC	5mg
Oxycodone: PO	6.6mg
Tramadol: PO	100mg

When adjusting a patient's regular pain relief medication remember to adjust the breakthrough medication dose too. The dose of the breakthrough medication should be ⅙ of the total regular medication taken in 24 hours.

- Consider topical analgesia
- Avoid mixing opiates
- Consider neuropathic agents
- Anxiety can make pain worse

Additional symptom management[4]

As a person approaches the end of their life, additional symptoms may arise.

These symptoms are listed below, along with medications that can be used to manage them, and their route of administration.

Excessive respiratory secretions

- Hyoscine hydrobromide 400mcg SC every 4 hours.
- Hyoscine butylbromide 20mg SC every 4 hours.
- Glycopyrronium bromide 200mcg SC every 4 hours.

Anorexia

- Prednisolone 15–30mg PO once daily, with gastric lining protection such as lansoprazole 15mg PO once daily.

Nausea and vomiting

- Cyclizine 50mg every 8 hours PO/SC/IM. This can be used to treat nausea and vomiting associated with gastric causes, raised intracranial pressure or secondary to medication.
- Metoclopramide 10mg PO/SC/IM every 8 hours. This is a prokinetic agent and can be used to treat gastric causes of nausea and vomiting such as bowel obstruction or stasis.
- Other agents which can be used are:
    - levomepromazine 6mg PO or 6.25mg SC as required
    - prochlorperazine 5mg PO every 8 hours or 3mg sublingually every 12 hours
    - ondansetron 8mg PO every 12 hours
    - haloperidol 1.5mg PO every 12 hours or 2.5–10mg SC over 24 hours.

Agitation

- Haloperidol 0.75–1.5mg SC/IM every 8 hours.
- Levomepromazine 6.25mg SC/IM every 2 hours.
- Lorazepam 0.5–1.0mg PO every 6 hours.
- Midazolam 2.5–5.0mg SC every 4–6 hours.

Bowel colic

- Hyoscine butylbromide 20mg SC every 8 hours.

Raised ICP and headaches

- Dexamethasone 16mg PO daily in divided doses and reduce after 5 days.

Other medications

- Laxatives, loperamide, antihistamines, anti-epileptics and benzodiazepines can also play a role in managing symptoms as they arise.

Syringe drivers

Syringe drivers (*Fig. 23.1*) are not always used to manage symptoms in patients who are at the end of their life; they can be used to treat a variety of conditions where enteral medication may be inappropriate or cannot be taken.

The aim is to provide continuous medication subcutaneously for patients who are unable to take medication via another route or for patients who require frequent injections.

Ideally no more than three different drugs should be added to one syringe, as there is a risk of drug precipitation.

Medication is usually dissolved in water, so it is important to prescribe water ampoules for injections when prescribing any drugs for a syringe driver.

Drug indications and associated medications are listed below[4].

For pain relief

- Calculate the total oral opiate dose (regular plus breakthrough) taken by the patient in 24 hours and convert this to oral morphine sulphate.
- The total oral morphine sulphate dose should then be converted to subcutaneous morphine sulphate (½ of total oral morphine dose) or subcutaneous diamorphine (⅓ of total oral morphine dose).
- This should be administered subcutaneously over 24 hours via the syringe driver.
- If the patient is opiate naïve then an appropriate starting range would be 5–10mg morphine sulphate or 2.5–5.0mg diamorphine over 24 hours.

For nausea

- Cyclizine 50–150mg or metoclopramide 20–30mg over 24 hours.

For agitation

- Haloperidol 5–30mg (this can also be used to manage nausea), midazolam 5–30mg (this can also be used to manage convulsions).

For secretions

- Hyoscine hydrobromide 1.2–2.0mg/24hrs or glycopyrronium bromide 0.6–1.2mg/24hrs.

For bowel colic

- Hyoscine hydrobromide 1.2–2.0mg/24hrs or hyoscine butylbromide 60mg/24hrs.

A typical starting regime for a syringe driver would consist of:

- Diamorphine 5.0mg
- Haloperidol 5.0mg
- Hyoscine hydrobromide 1.2mg

in 20ml of water over 24 hours

Feature recognition

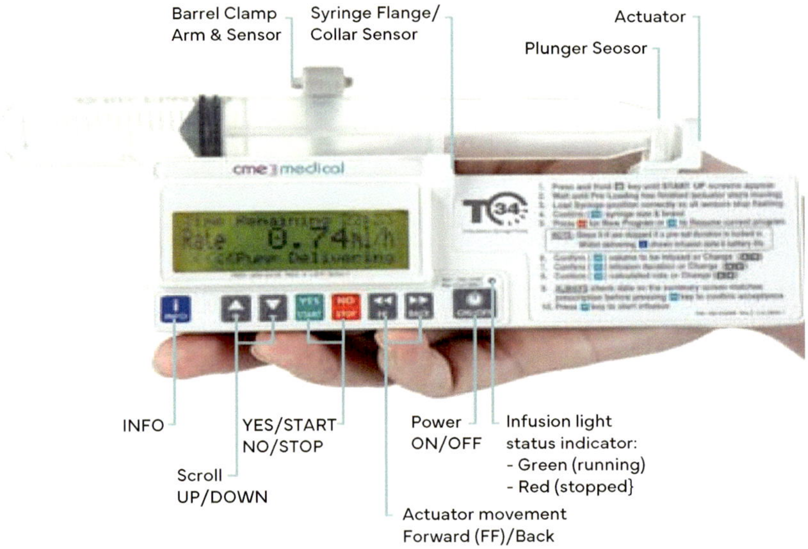

Fig. 23.1: A McKinley T34 syringe driver.

This is usually set up by the district nurses once medication has been prescribed. Reproduced from www.shropscommunityhealth.nhs.uk/content/doclib/10782.pdf under an Open Government Licence.

Prescribing syringe drivers

- It is good practice to prescribe a range for medications in a syringe driver, e.g. morphine sulphate 5–20mg/24hrs, as this allows the district nurses to titrate up the medication based on the patient's needs.
- Diamorphine can be mixed with cyclizine, dexamethasone, haloperidol, hyoscine hydrobromide, hyoscine butylbromide, levomepromazine, metoclopramide and midazolam.
- When seeing a patient in an OOH setting or at home, the process of authorising and arranging a syringe driver will involve administering a stat dose to control symptoms (stock may be available in the car), leaving an FP10 prescription for ampoules for medication and water to set up a syringe driver, filling in the district nurse forms (syringe driver section and just in case medication section) and requesting a district nurse visit to set up the syringe driver (the drivers are usually available to district nurses).

Liaising with family members and next of kin

- Be compassionate, considerate and empathetic.
- Always inform loved ones and the family of the process and what your intentions are; explain to them that your aim is to keep their loved one as comfortable as possible.
- Advise them that they can always call you back should they have any concerns or queries.

Summary for cancer/palliative care

- End of life care should be planned in advance, and appropriate resources and medication should be prescribed to minimise any distress to the patient and family.
- Don't forget to titrate up breakthrough analgesia when increasing the patient's regular analgesia.
- Avoid prescribing different types of opiates together, as there is an increased risk of respiratory depression.
- Ensure the patient and family have as much support as available.
- Avoid adding more than three drugs to the syringe driver as there is a risk of drug precipitation.
- Take into account the family and loved ones' wishes.
- Reassure the family that they can call back if there are any concerns.

References

1. NICE (2015) *Care of dying adults in the last days of life* [NG31]. Available at: www.nice.org.uk/guidance/ng31

2. NICE (revised 2023) *Palliative care – general issues*. Available at: https://cks.nice.org.uk/palliative-care-general-issues#!topicSummary

3. Royal College of General Practitioners (2020) *End of life and palliative care toolkit*. Available at: https://elearning.rcgp.org.uk/mod/book/view.php?id=12529

4. BNF (no date) *Prescribing in palliative care*. Available at: https://bnf.nice.org.uk/guidance/prescribing-in-palliative-care.html

24

Chapter 24: **Safeguarding and non-accidental injury**

SAFEGUARDING

"Safeguarding the rights of others is the most noble and beautiful end of a human being."
Khalil Gibran

Assessment of vulnerable patients and those with safeguarding concerns

Telephone

- Take a detailed history.
- Access summary care records and previous encounters.
- Assess capacity.
- Speak to the patient's carer or guardian if necessary.

If there are any concerns with regard to safeguarding, a face-to-face assessment should be undertaken.

Safeguarding

- Safeguarding is the term used to describe the process put in place to protect vulnerable adults and children from harm or potential harm and to protect their human rights[1],[2].
- Safeguarding is everyone's responsibility.
- Any person – especially a healthcare professional – who comes into contact with a vulnerable adult or a child has a duty to ensure the vulnerable person or child is protected from harm.
- The Children Act 2004 and The Care Act 2014 have put in place legislative processes and a framework to ensure this happens[3].
- If you suspect a child or vulnerable adult is at risk then you should raise your concerns in accordance with polices put in place by your employing organisation.
- All healthcare professionals in the UK should have regular safeguarding training.
- There should be policies and protocols in place, along with a safeguarding lead for every organisation in the NHS.
- Local councils will have safeguarding boards in place and their contact details should be readily available to raise any concerns.

- If a child or vulnerable adult is at immediate risk of harm, the emergency services should be informed.
- It is beyond the scope of this book to go into detail on safeguarding; however, important links are presented at the end of the chapter and it is essential all healthcare professionals are aware of and up to date with safeguarding training and policies.

Summary for safeguarding

- Safeguarding is everyone's responsibility.
- Raise concerns with a senior clinician or in accordance with your organisation's policy.

References

1. NHS England (no date) *Safeguarding*. Available at: www.england.nhs.uk/safeguarding/

2. Care Quality Commission (updated 2022) *Safeguarding people*. Available at: www.cqc.org.uk/what-we-do/how-we-do-our-job/safeguarding-people

3. UK Government (no date) *Safeguarding and social care for children*. Available at: www.gov.uk/childcare-parenting/safeguarding-and-social-care-for-children

NON-ACCIDENTAL INJURY

"Children are the world's most valuable resource and its best hope for the future."

John F. Kennedy

Assessment of children and patients with non-accidental injury

- All children and vulnerable adults suspected of having a non-accidental injury (NAI) should be assessed face-to-face by a competent clinician.
- The history and examination findings should be documented accurately.
- Discussion with the safeguarding teams should take place as soon as possible.
- Children should be discussed with the on-call paediatric team.
- If the patient is at immediate risk, inform the police.

Non-accidental injury [1],[2]

- Children will often present in an urgent care or OOH setting with injuries.
- It is important to check previous records; often organisations will have markers on the records of vulnerable adults and children who are subject to a protection or safeguarding plan.
- It is essential that all clinicians involved in assessing children and vulnerable adults are aware of the features of NAI.
- If NAI is suspected a thorough assessment is mandatory. This should include a full history and examination, along with any photographs of injuries and any relevant investigations.
- The following factors should lead to the suspicion of NAI:
  - a delay in presentation
  - discrepancies in the history
  - an absent history
  - clinical findings inconsistent with the history
  - repetitive injuries
  - unusual parental behaviour or mood
  - disclosure by the child or a witness
  - unusual demeanour or behaviour of the child.
- Sites of injury normally associated with NAI are:
  - face
  - chest wall
  - abdomen
  - genitalia
  - inner and outer thighs
  - buttocks
  - multiple site involvement.
- Bilateral retinal haemorrhages are strongly suggestive of non-accidental injury and can occur due to chest injuries, asphyxia, coagulation disorders, sepsis, meningitis, trauma to the cranium and severe shaking, as well as during normal birth.
- Sites commonly associated with accidental injury are bony prominences, the shins and the front of the body.
- The most common cause of traumatic death in paediatric patients is intracranial injury.
- Trauma to the cranium can result in subdural and extradural haematomas, ischaemic encephalopathy and intracranial haemorrhages. These can lead to loss of consciousness, seizures, a tense fontanelle, apnoea and death.
- Injury to the major organs is the second most common cause of death in infants subjected to physical abuse.
- The presentation of the child will be dependent on the time elapsed since the injury.
- Chronic injuries can result in poor feeding and failure to thrive.
- Certain conditions can mimic NAI; for example, blistering of the skin from non-accidental burn injuries can often resemble vesicular lesions seen in impetigo, chickenpox and shingles.
- Other conditions may also contribute to genuine accidental injuries, such as haemophilia, severe anaemia and brittle bone disease.

- Children suspected of having NAI should be discussed with the on-call paediatrician and safeguarding lead for the area.

Features suggestive of NAI in children[3]

- Delayed presentation
- Inconsistent or absent history
- Inconsistent clinical findings
- Repetitive injuries
- Unusual parental behaviour or mood
- Unusual child behaviour or demeanour
- Disclosure by the child or witness

Sites of injury associated with NAI[3]

- Face
- Chest wall
- Abdomen
- Genitalia
- Inner and outer thighs
- Buttocks
- Multiple sites

Summary for non-accidental injury

- Consider NAI in all children and vulnerable adults who present with injuries.
- A full history and examination is mandatory.
- Raise concerns with a senior clinician or in accordance with your organisation's policy.

References

1. Cawson, P., Wattam, C., Brooker, S. and Kelly, G. (2000) *Child Maltreatment in the UK: a study of prevalence of child abuse and neglect*. NSPCC.

2. Bhupal, H.K. (2016) *Clinical Forensic & Legal Medicine: MCQ's, answers and explanatory notes* (Child abuse and non-accidental injury, pp. 11–19). CreateSpace Independent Publishing Platform.

3. Royal College of Paediatrics and Child Health (2015) *The Physical Signs of Child Sexual Abuse: an evidence-based review and guidance for best practice*. Available at: www.rcpch.ac.uk/shop-publications/physical-signs-child-sexual-abuse-evidence-based-review

25

Chapter 25: **Basic life support**

"You may never know what results come of your actions, but if you do nothing there will be no results."
Mahatma Gandhi

Assessing a collapsed person

- Always ensure it is safe to approach someone who has collapsed.
- Call for help.
- Assess breathing and circulation for 10 seconds.
- If the collapsed person is breathing and has a palpable pulse, place them in the recovery position (*Fig. 25.2*) and ensure help is on the way.
- Consider checking basic observations such as pulse, blood pressure, oxygen saturations, temperature and blood glucose.
- If heart and breath sounds are absent, begin basic life support as described below.

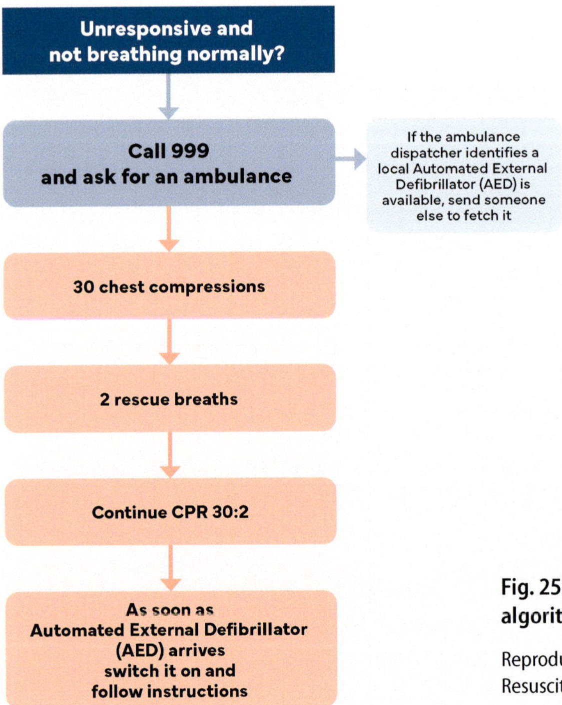

Fig. 25.1: Adult basic life support algorithm.

Reproduced with the kind permission of Resuscitation Council UK.

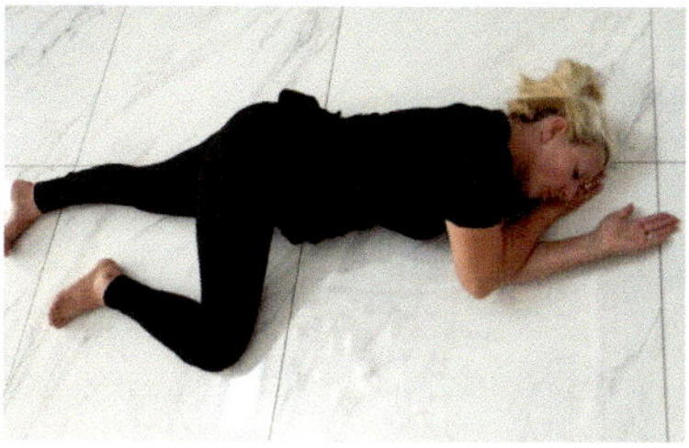

Fig. 25.2: Recovery position – notice the right hand placed under the head and also the right leg across the left leg.

Below is the detailed sequence of steps if an AED is available[1].

Sequence	Technical description
SAFETY	**Make sure you, the collapsed person and any bystanders are safe**
RESPONSE	**Check the person for a response** • Gently shake the shoulders and ask loudly: *"Are you all right?"* • If the person responds, leave them in the position in which you found them, provided there is no further danger; try to find out what is wrong with them and get help if needed; reassess them regularly.
AIRWAY	**Open the airway** • Turn the person onto their back. • Place your hand on their forehead and gently tilt the head back; with your fingertips under the point of their chin, lift the chin to open the airway.
BREATHING	**Look, listen and feel for normal breathing for no more than 10 seconds** In the first few minutes after cardiac arrest, a person may be barely breathing, or taking infrequent, slow and noisy gasps. Do not confuse this with normal breathing. If you have any doubt whether breathing is normal, act as if the person is not breathing normally and prepare to start CPR.
CALL 999	**Call an ambulance (999)** • Ask a helper to call if possible, otherwise call them yourself. • Stay with the collapsed person when making the call, if possible. • Activate the speaker function on the phone to aid communication with the ambulance service.
SEND FOR AED	**Send someone to get an AED if available** If you are on your own, do not leave the person, start CPR.

Continues overleaf

<table>
<tr><th>Sequence</th><th>Technical description</th></tr>
<tr><td>CIRCULATION</td><td>Start chest compressions<ul><li>Kneel by the side of the person.</li><li>Place the heel of one hand in the centre of the person's chest (which is the lower half of the person's sternum).</li><li>Place the heel of your other hand on top of the first hand.</li><li>Interlock the fingers of your hands and ensure that pressure is not applied over the person's ribs.</li><li>Keep your arms straight.</li><li>Do not apply any pressure over the upper abdomen or the bottom end of the bony sternum.</li><li>Position your shoulders vertically above the person's chest and press down on the sternum to a depth of 5–6cm.</li><li>After each compression, release all the pressure on the chest without losing contact between your hands and the sternum.</li><li>Repeat at a rate of 100–120 compressions per minute.</li></ul></td></tr>
<tr><td>GIVE RESCUE BREATHS</td><td>After 30 compressions open the airway again using head tilt and chin lift and give 2 rescue breaths. If a face mask and bag are available use these, otherwise give rescue breaths manually.<ul><li>Pinch the soft part of the nose closed, using the index finger and thumb, resting your hand on the forehead.</li><li>Allow the mouth to open, but maintain chin lift.</li><li>Take a normal breath and place your lips around the person's mouth, making sure that you have a good seal.</li><li>Blow steadily into the mouth while watching for the chest to rise, taking about 1 second as in normal breathing; this is an effective rescue breath.</li><li>Maintaining head tilt and chin lift, take your mouth away from the person and watch for the chest to fall as air comes out.</li><li>Take another normal breath and blow into the person's mouth once more to achieve a total of two effective rescue breaths. Do not interrupt compressions by more than 10 seconds to deliver two breaths. Then return your hands without delay to the correct position on the sternum and give a further 30 chest compressions.</li></ul>Continue with chest compressions and rescue breaths in a ratio of 30:2.

If you are untrained or unable to do rescue breaths, give chest compression only CPR.</td></tr>
</table>

Sequence	Technical description
IF AN AED ARRIVES	**Switch on the AED** • Attach the electrode pads on the person's bare chest. • If more than one rescuer is present, CPR should be continued while electrode pads are being attached to the chest. • Follow the spoken or visual directions. • Ensure that nobody is touching the collapsed person while the AED is analysing the rhythm. **If a shock is indicated, deliver shock** • Ensure that nobody is touching the collapsed person. • Push shock button as directed (fully automatic AEDs will deliver the shock automatically). • Immediately restart CPR at a ratio of 30:2. • Continue as directed by the voice or visual prompts. **If no shock is indicated, continue CPR** • Immediately resume CPR. • Continue as directed by the voice or visual prompts.
CONTINUE CPR	**Do not interrupt resuscitation until:** • A health professional tells you to stop. • You become exhausted. • The person is definitely waking up, moving, opening eyes and breathing normally. It is rare for CPR alone to restart the heart. Unless you are certain the person has recovered, continue CPR.

Continues overleaf

Sequence	Technical description
RECOVERY POSITION	**If you are certain the person is breathing normally but is still unresponsive, place in the recovery position** • Remove the person's glasses, if worn. • Kneel beside the person and make sure that both their legs are straight. • Place the arm nearest to you out at right angles to the body, elbow bent with the hand palm-up. • Bring the far arm across the chest, and hold the back of the hand against the collapsed person's cheek nearest to you. • With your other hand, grasp the far leg just above the knee and pull it up, keeping the foot on the ground. • Keeping the person's hand pressed against their cheek, pull on the far leg to roll the person towards you onto their side. • Adjust the upper leg so that both the hip and knee are bent at right angles. • Tilt the head back to make sure that the airway remains open. • If necessary, adjust the hand under the cheek to keep the head tilted and facing downwards to allow liquid material to drain from the mouth. • Check breathing regularly. **Be prepared to restart CPR immediately if the person deteriorates or stops breathing normally.**

Choking

Below is the sequence of steps to manage someone who is choking[1]:

Sequence	Technical description
SUSPECT CHOKING	**Be alert to choking, particularly if the person is eating**
ENCOURAGE TO COUGH	**Instruct the person to cough**
GIVE BACK BLOWS	**If the cough is ineffective give up to five back blows** • Stand to the side and slightly behind the person. • Support the chest with one hand and lean the person well forwards so that when the obstructing object is dislodged it comes out of the mouth rather than goes further down the airway. • Give five sharp blows between the shoulder blades with the heel of your other hand.

Sequence	Technical description
GIVE ABDOMINAL THRUSTS	**If back blows are ineffective give up to five abdominal thrusts** • Stand behind the person and put both arms round the upper part of the abdomen. • Lean the person forwards. • Clench your fist and place it between the umbilicus (navel) and the ribcage. • Grasp this hand with your other hand and pull sharply inwards and upwards. • Repeat up to five times. • If the obstruction is still not relieved, continue alternating five back blows with five abdominal thrusts.
START CPR	**Start CPR if the person becomes unresponsive** • Support the person carefully to the ground. • Immediately call or ask someone to call the ambulance service. • Begin CPR with chest compressions.

Anaphylaxis and allergic reactions

Presentation

- Anaphylaxis is a severe life-threatening generalised or systemic hypersensitivity reaction.
- There can be various triggers including animal stings, foods, medication and cosmetic products.
- Patients may or may not have a rash.
- The affected person may have dyspnoea, facial swelling and tongue swelling.
- Continued histamine release will result in vasodilation, hypotension and collapse.

Assessment

- There will be tachycardia, tachypnoea, low oxygen saturations, stridor and later on hypovolaemia, indicating anaphylactic shock.

Management[2]

- All patients with anaphylaxis should be given immediate basic life support and the following:
  - high-flow oxygen
  - intravenous fluids
  - chlorphenamine 10mg IM
  - hydrocortisone 100–200mg IM
  - adrenaline IM (150mcg for children under 5 years, 300mcg for children aged 5–11 years, 500mcg for adults).

Anaphylaxis?

A = Airway **B** = Breathing **C** = Circulation **D** = Disability **E** = Exposure

Diagnosis – look for:

- Sudden onset of Airway and/or Breathing and/or Circulation problems[1]
- And usually skin changes (e.g. itchy rash)

Call for HELP

Call resuscitation team or ambulance

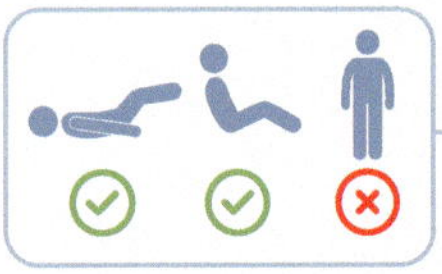

- Remove trigger if possible (e.g. stop any infusion)
- Lie patient flat (with or without legs elevated)
  - A sitting position may make breathing easier
  - If pregnant, lie on left side

Give intramuscular (IM) adrenaline[2]

Inject at **anterolateral aspect** – middle third of the thigh

- Establish airway
- Give high flow oxygen
- Apply monitoring: pulse oximetry, ECG, blood pressure

If no response:

- Repeat IM adrenaline after 5 minutes
- IV fluid bolus[3]

If no improvement in Breathing or Circulation problems[1] despite TWO doses of IM adrenaline:

- Confirm resuscitation team or ambulance has been called
- Follow REFRACTORY ANAPHYLAXIS ALGORITHM

1. Life-threatening problems

Airway
Hoarse voice, stridor

Breathing
↑work of breathing, wheeze, fatigue, cyanosis, SpO_2 <94%

Circulation
Low blood pressure, signs of shock, confusion, reduced consciousness

2. Intramuscular (IM) adrenaline

Use adrenaline at 1 mg/mL (1:1000) concentration

Adult and child >12 years:	500 micrograms IM (0.5 mL)
Child 6–12 years:	300 micrograms IM (0.3 mL)
Child 6 months to 6 years:	150 micrograms IM (0.15 mL)
Child <6 months:	100–150 micrograms IM (0.1–0.15 mL)

The above doses are for IM injection **only**.
Intravenous adrenaline for anaphylaxis to be given **only by experienced specialists** in an appropriate setting.

3. IV fluid challenge

Use crystalloid

Adults: 500–1000 mL
Children: 10 mL/kg

Fig. 25.3: Anaphylaxis algorithm.

Reproduced with the kind permission of Resuscitation Council UK.

- Adrenaline should be injected into the anterolateral aspect of the middle third of the thigh.
- The dose can be repeated after 5 minutes but should be administered into the contralateral thigh, as vasoconstriction from the first dose can reduce absorption of the second dose.
- The patient should be referred to ED via ambulance immediately.

Summary for basic life support

- It is good practice to have BLS refresher training every 6–12 months.
- Ensure you are familiar with the location of the resuscitation equipment and how to alert colleagues.
- Always inject the repeat dose of adrenaline into the contralateral thigh.

References

1. Resuscitation Council UK (2021) *Adult basic life support guidelines*. Available at: www.resus.org.uk/library/2021-resuscitation-guidelines/adult-basic-life-support-guidelines

2. Resuscitation Council UK (2021) *Emergency treatment of anaphylactic reactions: guidelines for healthcare providers*. Available at: www.resus.org.uk/library/additional-guidance/guidance-anaphylaxis/emergency-treatment

26

Chapter 26: **Managing abnormal blood test results**

"Blood is a juice of rarest quality."
Johann Wolfgang von Goethe

- It is not uncommon to receive abnormal blood test results in an OOH setting. This often occurs when a patient has had a blood sample taken during the day, and the GP surgery has closed by the time the results are available. As a result, the laboratory will often pass these abnormal blood test results on to the OOH GP service to assess and act upon.
- It is impossible to cover **all** blood test results in this book; indeed, there are other books available which do this. However, it is possible to provide the most common blood test results that the OOH GP service is asked to assess.
- With any single result it is helpful to find out why the patient had blood tests done (often the laboratory will have the clinical indication recorded on the request form) and to find out about previous blood test results. Speaking to the laboratory technician directly is often an option and their contact number is usually provided with the results.
- Further information may be obtained by checking the patient's summary care record (SCR) or patient medical record (PMR). This should be done after requesting permission from the patient or, if you are unable to contact the patient, it is in the patient's best interests.
- In the majority of cases patients can be assessed over the phone and a clinical management decision can be made; only rarely will patients require a face-to-face appointment.
- In cases where it is not possible to get hold of the patient, it is prudent to phone local emergency departments to enquire whether the patient has been admitted to hospital, or even make a home visit to check on them.

HAEMATOLOGY

Haemoglobin (normal range: adult male: 130–180g/L; adult female: 115–165g/L)

Introduction

Haemoglobin (Hb) is a protein found in blood cells which is responsible for carrying oxygen around the body.

- A gradual decrease in Hb (over months) can be tolerated relatively well by most people who do not have any comorbidities. On a few occasions I have seen patients with a Hb of less than 80g/L who have been asymptomatic. Conversely, a sudden drop in Hb, even by a few g/L, can produce symptoms.
- As with any anaemia, it is important to identify whether it is a microcytic, normocytic or macrocytic anaemia:
  - microcytic anaemia is commonly seen with iron deficiency and blood loss
  - normocytic anaemia is commonly seen in people with chronic diseases such as chronic kidney disease
  - macrocytic anaemia is found in patients who have low vitamin B12 and/or folate levels.

Assessment

- When presented with an unexpected low Hb or a significantly low Hb (<100g/L) result, it is essential to call the patient.
- Take a clear history as to the reason for the blood test.
- Enquire about symptoms of anaemia including fatigue, shortness of breath, palpitations, chest pain, light-headedness, episodes of pre-syncope and syncope.
- Ask about any active blood loss or occult bleeding, e.g. melaena, excessive vaginal bleeding.
- Take a detailed medication history; patients on anticoagulants are more likely to haemorrhage.
- Find out if there is someone with the patient.

Management

- In general, patients who are asymptomatic, with no active bleeding, with a gradual Hb drop and a Hb not lower than 80g/L, can be referred back to their own GP the following day.
- Patients who are symptomatic and/or have active bleeding should be referred to ED or the on-call medical team.

Neutrophils (normal range: 1.5–8.0 × 10^9/L)

Introduction
Neutrophils play a vital role in fighting off bacterial infection.

Results: <1.5 × 10^9/L = neutropenia[1]
- A low neutrophil count can make patients more susceptible to bacterial infections and neutropenic sepsis.
- Causes of neutropenia include:
  - benign ethnic neutropenia (in Afro-Caribbeans, Arabs and those with Jewish ancestry)
  - chemotherapy
  - aplastic anaemia
  - leukaemias and bone marrow disorders
  - infections
  - drugs (quinidine, cephalosporins, sulphonamides, penicillins and hydralazine)
  - autoimmune conditions (rheumatoid arthritis, inflammatory bowel disease, autoimmune hepatitis, Hodgkin's lymphoma)[1].

Assessment
- Speak to the laboratory technician and determine the indication for the blood test. Also ascertain what previous levels were; has there been a gradual drop, or has it been sudden?
- Speak to the patient on the phone with the aim of establishing how unwell they may be.
- There may be a history of recurrent infections or frequent antibiotic usage.

Red flag features

Any symptoms suggestive of infection (such as pyrexia and rigors), sore throat, productive cough, shortness of breath, diarrhoea, vomiting, abdominal pain, chest pain, confusion, rashes, dysuria and non-healing wounds.

Management
- Patients who have mild and stable neutropenia without any red flag features can be referred back to their own GP the following day.
- Provide advice on red flag features to look out for and advise the patient to call back if they have any concerns.
- Ensure there will be someone with the patient overnight.
- Patients with neutropenia and features suggestive of an active infection should be referred immediately to the on-call medical team; consider an emergency ambulance transfer to hospital[2].

Results: >8.0 × 10^9/L = neutrophilia

Causes of neutrophilia include:
- pregnancy (benign and transient – this does not require any intervention)
- infections

- inflammatory conditions (such as gout and rheumatoid arthritis)
- burns
- myocardial infarction
- smoking (chronic and stable neutrophilia)
- excessive and/or strenuous exercise
- drugs (such as corticosteroids)
- neoplastic and myeloproliferative disorders (such as acute myeloid leukaemia)[3].

Assessment

- When assessing an abnormal blood test result of neutrophilia, speak to the laboratory technician and determine previous levels as well as the background history of the patient (or check the patient's SCR or PMR).
- If speaking to the patient on the phone determine if they are clinically unwell, e.g. have pyrexia, dyspnoea, rigors.
- The aim is to make a decision on whether the patient needs to be admitted to hospital immediately.

Management

- Patients with chronic neutrophilia, such as seen in smokers or those on long-term oral corticosteroid therapy, can be followed up by their own GP.
- Patients with an elevated neutrophil count who are describing a focus of infection and are not on any antibiotics may benefit from a face-to-face appointment. This would be to perform a physical assessment, confirm the source of infection and to prescribe appropriate antibiotics.
- Patients who are describing features of sepsis or an acute myeloproliferative disorder (dyspnoea, bruising, bleeding, bone pain, night sweats, weight loss)[4] should be referred to the on-call medical team. Consider a blue light ambulance transfer for these patients.

Lymphocytes (normal range: 1.0–4.0 × 10^9/L)

Introduction

Lymphocytes play a role in fighting infections, predominantly viral infections.

Results

- It is uncommon for abnormal lymphocyte counts to be referred to the OOH GP service. In most cases changes develop gradually and patients will be clinically well.
- **Lymphopenia** (<1.0 × 10^9/L) can be caused by viral infections such as the common cold, HIV, autoimmune conditions (such as SLE, rheumatoid arthritis), severe stress, prolonged exercise, chemotherapy and bone marrow disorders.
- **Lymphocytosis** (>4.0 × 10^9/L) can be caused by infections (viral, protozoal, tuberculosis), lymphoma, chronic lymphocytic leukaemia (CLL) and acute lymphoblastic leukaemia (ALL).

Assessment and management

- It is important to determine the medical history of the patient and to enquire about previous results.

- Patients who are well on the phone and are asymptomatic can be referred back to their own GP the next working day.
- Patients with features of a viral infection who are systemically well can also be referred back to their doctor, as can patients with CLL.
- Patients with features suggestive of ALL, such as generalised fatigue, anaemia, lethargy, confusion, weight loss, bone pain, bleeding, bruising and petechiae, or those who are systemically unwell, should be referred to the on-call medical team.

Platelets (normal range: 150–450 × 10^9/L)

Introduction

Platelets play a vital role in the coagulation of blood.

Results

Thrombocytosis (>450 × 10^9/L) refers to elevated platelet levels.

- This can be found in infective or inflammatory processes.
- Persistently high levels are considered to be a soft marker for cancer.

Thrombocytopenia (<150 × 10^9/L) refers to reduced platelet levels, commonly divided into:
    - mild: >100 × 10^9/L
    - moderate: 50–100 × 10^9/L
    - severe: <50 × 10^9/L.
- There are various causes of thrombocytopenia, including splenomegaly, hepatomegaly, excessive alcohol intake, pregnancy, infections such as malaria, medications such as heparin, and dilutional, e.g. post transfusion.
- The risk of haemorrhage is greatly increased when platelet levels drop below 20 × 10^9/L [5].

Assessment

- When assessing patients with thrombocytopenia, enquire about features suggestive of bleeding:
    - spontaneous bruising
    - petechiae
    - haemoptysis
    - epistaxis
    - retinal haemorrhages
    - pallor
    - acute painful joint deformities.

Management

- In an OOH setting, patients with thrombocytosis will not require admission or referral to hospital and can be followed up by their own GP the following day. Persistent thrombocytosis is considered a 'soft' marker for neoplastic disease, and this should be taken into consideration when the patient is assessed by their own GP.
- Patients with thrombocytopenia and any of the above features on assessment should be referred immediately to the on-call medical team.

D-dimer (adult normal value: <500ng/ml)

Introduction

The D-dimer is a protein fragment that is released into the bloodstream when a blood clot breaks down.

- A D-dimer blood test is commonly requested to exclude a DVT (and rarely a PE, although patients with a suspected PE should be referred to hospital for a CTPA).
- Although the D-dimer blood test is highly sensitive it has a low specificity [6] with a number of conditions causing it to be elevated, including pregnancy, infections, cancer, injuries and recent surgery.

Presentation

- In my experience, clinicians will often request a D-dimer when there is lower limb swelling, to exclude a DVT. However, lower limb swelling can be caused by cellulitis and a D-dimer will often be elevated in infections, so an elevated D-dimer may just complicate the picture.
- Nonetheless, a negative D-dimer can be helpful in ruling out thromboembolic disease rather than a positive one confirming it.

Assessment and management

- A DVT can be a potentially life-threatening condition; the clot can break off and result in a fatal PE.
- Patients who have a high D-dimer with symptoms suggestive of a DVT should be referred to their local ED or DVT clinic.
- Although duplex ultrasound scans (used to confirm or rule out a DVT) will usually not be available out of normal working hours, the patient can be started on low molecular weight heparin as a precaution and be brought back for a scan in normal working hours.

International normalised ratio

Introduction

The international normalised ratio (INR) is used to measure the time taken for blood to clot. The higher the INR, the longer it will take for blood to clot and the higher the risk of haemorrhage.

Presentation

- There are various conditions in which an elevated INR is preferable (where there is an increased risk of developing blood clots):
  - having a prosthetic heart valve
  - if the heart is in atrial fibrillation.
- The target INR is dependent on the condition being treated.
- Warfarin is a drug used to thin the blood and increase the clotting (and hence INR) time.
- The INR blood test is used to monitor the blood's response to warfarin and to determine the warfarin dose, which varies according to the INR.
- With the advent of DOACs (direct oral anticoagulants) and the slow phasing out of warfarin, having to deal with elevated INR levels in an OOH setting is becoming less and less common.

Assessment

- When assessing a patient with a high INR, take a detailed history over the phone.
- Enquire about the indication for warfarin, comorbidities and additional medication.
- Ask about previous INR results and also warfarin dosages.
- The key is to determine if the patient has active bleeding; features that suggest this would be:
  - spontaneous bruising
  - petechiae
  - haemoptysis
  - epistaxis
  - retinal haemorrhages
  - haematemesis
  - rectal haemorrhage
  - haematuria
  - pallor
  - acute painful joint deformities.

Management

- Patients with features of active bleeding should be referred to ED immediately – consider arranging a blue light ambulance.
- Patients who are stable with an elevated INR should be advised to stop taking their warfarin, avoid any activities that put them at risk of bleeding, and to follow up with the warfarin clinic or their own GP the following day.
- Advise the patient that at the first sign of bleeding they should call 111 or the OOH GP service, or attend their nearest ED.

Random plasma glucose levels (normal range: 4.0–11.1mmol/L)

Presentation

- Random plasma glucose levels carry very little diagnostic value and are now rarely requested. Very occasionally the laboratory may forward you a very low or a very high plasma glucose value.

Assessment

- In each case, determine whether the result is a true random sample or if the patient was fasting.
- Ascertain whether the patient is diabetic.
- By the time the result has been made available to you several hours will have passed, so phone the patient and determine if they are acutely unwell.
- Diabetic patients may be able to check their blood glucose whilst you are talking to them.

Management

- The majority of patients can be followed up by their own GP the following day. Patients who have persistently high blood glucose or are acutely unwell should be discussed with the on-call medical team.

ELECTROLYTE IMBALANCES

Hyperkalaemia (serum potassium of >5.5mmol/L; normal range 3.5–5.5mmol/L)

Presentation

- Hyperkalaemia refers to raised potassium levels in the serum and this can be caused by:
  - medications such as ACE inhibitors and potassium-sparing diuretics (e.g. spironolactone)
  - kidney disease
  - major trauma or crush injuries
  - rhabdomyolysis
  - Addison's disease
  - haemolysis of red blood cells as a result of blood samples not being processed in time.
- Often patients with hyperkalaemia will be asymptomatic; however:
  - mildly high levels (5.5–5.9mmol/L) can cause symptoms such as fatigue, nausea and myalgia
  - moderately high levels (6.0–6.4mmol/L) can cause abdominal pain, vomiting, muscular cramps and weakness
  - high levels (above 6.5mmol/L) can cause sudden palpitations, chest pain, dyspnoea and sudden cardiac arrest [7].

Assessment

- Call the laboratory and find out about previous potassium levels and whether the patient has a history of chronic kidney disease.
- The patient's SCR will also provide information including any medications which may have contributed to a raised potassium.
- Speak to the patient and enquire about any symptoms.

Management

- Patients with mildly elevated potassium levels who are asymptomatic should be advised to withhold any medication that may be contributing to raised potassium levels and also to avoid foods rich in potassium, such as dried fruits, leafy green vegetables, legumes and fish.
- They should be advised to follow up with their GP the following day.
- Patients with a raised potassium who are symptomatic or those with a moderately high level and above should be referred to ED or the on-call medical team for a repeat blood test, ECG and further management.
- ECG changes seen in hyperkalaemia include a flat P-wave, prolonged PR interval, prolonged QRS duration, a tall T-wave. Severe hyperkalaemia can result in bradycardia, arrhythmias and asystole.

Hypokalaemia (serum potassium of <3.5mmol/L; normal range 3.5–5.5mmol/L)

Presentation

- This is a relatively uncommon presentation in an OOH setting.

- Common causes include:
  - chronic kidney disease
  - diarrhoea
  - vomiting
  - laxative abuse
  - diuretics
  - hyperaldosteronism.
- Classification of hypokalaemia is as follows:
  - mild hypokalaemia is 3.1–3.4mmol/L
  - moderate hypokalaemia is 2.5–3.0mmol/L
  - severe hypokalaemia is <2.5mmol/L [8].

Assessment

- Symptoms to check for include fatigue, myalgia, muscle cramps, abdominal pain, constipation, nausea and palpitations.

Management

- Patients with mild hypokalaemia who are asymptomatic can be advised to follow up with their own GP the following day. Their GP can investigate potential causes and initiate oral supplementation with potassium salts.
- Patients with moderate to severe hypokalaemia, or those who are symptomatic, should be referred to ED for further investigations and an ECG.

Hypernatraemia (>146mmol/L; normal range 133–146mmol/L)

Presentation

- Having to deal with hypernatraemia (raised sodium levels) is relatively uncommon in an OOH setting.
- Common causes include:
  - inadequate fluid intake
  - excessive fluid loss
  - chronic kidney disease
  - diabetes insipidus
  - medications such as diuretics, corticosteroids and lithium[9].

Assessment

- Patients can be asymptomatic and in the case of elderly patients, mild chronic hypernatraemia can exist.
- Symptoms include polydipsia, fatigue, muscle twitches, confusion and seizures.

Management

- Patients who are asymptomatic can be advised to follow up with their own GP the following day.
- Patients who are symptomatic should be referred to their local ED.

Hyponatraemia (<135mmol/L; normal range 133–146mmol/L)

Presentation

- Hyponatraemia refers to low plasma sodium levels and can be categorised as follows:
  - mild (130–135mmol/L)
  - moderate (125–129mmol/L)
  - severe (<125 mmol/L)[10].
- Causes include:
  - hypovolaemia (severe vomiting, diarrhoea, bowel obstruction)
  - chronic kidney disease
  - chronic heart disease
  - hepatic impairment
  - SIADH (syndrome of inappropriate antidiuretic hormone)
  - surgery
  - polydipsia
  - Addison's disease (low sodium, high potassium, hypovolaemia)
  - medications, such as diuretics (e.g. thiazide) and antidepressants (e.g. SSRIs).
- Patients with mild chronic hyponatraemia tend to be asymptomatic and may have had this for years.
- Patients with acute or severe hyponatraemia may complain of fatigue, nausea, vomiting, headaches, confusion, irritability, muscle spasms and decreased urine output.
- Neurological symptoms such as paralysis and seizures can also occur.
- Patients who are hypovolaemic will have a low blood pressure, feel light-headed and may complain of pre-syncopal or syncopal episodes.

Assessment

- It is important to call the laboratory and determine previous sodium levels.
- On phoning patients with moderate to severe hyponatraemia, enquire about previous results and possible underlying causes.

Management

- If the hyponatraemia is mild and the patient is asymptomatic, advise the patient about increasing their oral salt intake and following up with their own GP the next day.
- Patients with moderate–severe hyponatraemia or with severe symptoms should be referred to their local ED.
- Very rarely will a face-to-face assessment be required to determine the patient's hydration status – in the majority of cases a plan of action can be determined via a telephone history.

OTHER BLOOD TESTS

Raised creatinine (>120mmol/L; normal range: 60–120mmol/L) and/or
low eGFR (<60ml/min/1.73m^2; normal range: 90–120ml/min/1.73m^2)

Presentation

- A raised creatinine and low eGFR (estimated glomerular filtration rate) indicate chronic kidney disease or an acute kidney injury.
- Chronic kidney disease (CKD) tends to develop insidiously, and patients will often have risk factors such as older age, diabetic nephropathy, hypertensive nephropathy, autoimmune conditions and glomerular diseases[11].
- Symptoms of CKD include anorexia, weight loss, oedema, fatigue, haematuria, reduced urine output, insomnia, generalised pruritus, muscle spasms, dyspnoea and chest pain.
- Acute kidney disease or injury (AKI) can also present with the above, but the onset tends to be acute.
- Causes of CKD are divided into:
    - pre-renal (hypovolaemia)
    - renal (damage to the kidney, e.g. from medication)
    - post-renal (obstruction of the urine outflow from the kidneys).
- AKI can be divided, as shown in *Table 26.1* [12]:

Table 26.1: Summary staging system for AKI in adults (based on the KDIGO classification)

Stage	Criteria
1	Creatinine rise of ≥26mmol/L within 48h *or* Creatinine rise of 50–99% from baseline within 7 days* (1.50–1.99 × baseline) *or* Urine output** less than 0.5ml/kg/h for more than 6h
2	100–199% creatinine rise from baseline within 7 days* (2.00–2.99 × baseline) *or* Urine output** less than 0.5ml/kg/h for more than 12h
3	≥200% or more creatinine rise from baseline within 7 days* (3.00 or more × baseline) *or* Creatinine rise to 354mmol/L or more with acute rise of 26mmol/L or more within 48h or 50% or more rise within 7 days *or* Urine output** less than 0.3ml/kg/h for 24h or anuria for 12h

* The rise is known (based on previous blood tests) or presumed (based on history) to have occurred within 7 days.
** Measurement of urine output may not be practical in primary care, but can be considered in a person with a catheter.
Adapted from: [13, 14]

Assessment

- In an OOH setting it is important to determine if this is acute, acute on chronic, or chronic.

- A phone call to the laboratory is usually necessary to determine previous eGFR levels. The patient's SCR or PMR may also include a diagnosis of CKD and have previous results listed.
- All patients should be assessed over the phone.
- The aim of the history is to determine the presence or absence of symptoms, to identify underlying causes and to gain a better understanding of previous results.
- Very rarely will a patient need to be seen face-to-face in an OOH setting, with the management plan evident from the history and blood test results.

Management

- Patients with Stage 1 AKI can be referred back to their own GP, provided there are no symptoms or acute underlying causes requiring treatment, and there are no electrolyte imbalances such as hyperkalaemia.
- Patients with Stage 2 AKI and above, symptoms of AKI, electrolyte imbalances (especially hyperkalaemia), or those requiring urgent treatment (e.g. urinary outflow obstruction, sepsis) should be referred to the on-call medical team.

C-reactive protein (normal range: 0–5mg/L)

Introduction

C-reactive protein (CRP) is a protein produced by the liver during the acute phase of an infection or inflammatory response.

Presentation

- Elevated levels are detected in blood plasma.
- It can be used to determine if there is an underlying infection or inflammation responsible for the patient's symptoms.
- It has a sensitivity of 84.3%, but it is quite non-specific (specificity of 46.15%) [15].
- Changes in CRP can be used to monitor recovery from infections or relapses of inflammatory conditions such as rheumatoid arthritis.

Assessment

- With all patients it is important to take a history.
- Although CRP levels can be quite high (often in the hundreds), patients may sound and appear reasonably well.
- When assessing a patient on the phone, the clinician needs to consider whether the patient should be referred to hospital immediately or whether the patient's GP can follow them up in the morning. It is important to consider previous CRP results; a decreasing CRP would suggest an improving clinical and biochemical picture.

Management

- In general, if the patient is clinically unwell then a referral to the on-call medical team is warranted.

Thyroid function tests

Presentation

- The most sensitive marker for thyroid function is thyroid-stimulating hormone (TSH). Normal levels are 0.4–4.0mU/L.
- TSH is released from the pituitary gland and has a negative feedback relationship with the thyroid gland.
- An elevated TSH level (>4.0mU/L) indicates hypothyroidism, and a low TSH (<0.4mU/L) indicates hyperthyroidism.

Assessment

- Patients may already have a history of thyroid dysfunction, and this may be mentioned on the blood test request form or evident from previous thyroid function test results.
- It is important to phone the patient and gather a relevant history, paying particular attention to **red flag symptoms such as palpitations, shortness of breath and chest pain**.
- These symptoms can arise due to thyroid overdrive or cardiac impairment secondary to hypothyroidism.

Management

- Referral to hospital is very rarely needed and most patients will be experiencing the symptoms of thyroid dysfunction for weeks and perhaps months.
- Most patients can be advised to follow up with their own GP the following day, but clearly the presence of red flags (although rare) would warrant a referral to the on-call medical team.

Liver function tests

Presentation

- Under stress the liver releases various enzymes into the bloodstream, including alanine transferase, alkaline phosphatases and gamma glutamyl transferase. Bilirubin levels can also be elevated.

Assessment

- It is important to gather as much information as possible by phoning the laboratory and enquiring about the reason for the blood tests and asking about previous results.
- Further information will be available on the patient's SCR or PMR.
- On speaking to the patient, take a detailed history, paying particular attention to reasons why the blood tests were requested.

Management

- Patients who are not acutely unwell or are asymptomatic can be followed up by their own GP the following day.
- Patients who sound acutely unwell, especially describing symptoms of infection (e.g. pyrexia) should be referred to the on-call medical team.

References

1. Justiz Vaillant, A.A., Rout, P., Reynolds, S.B. and Zito, P.M. (updated 2024) *Neutropenia*. StatPearls. Available at: www.ncbi.nlm.nih.gov/books/NBK507702

2. NICE (revised 2024) *Neutropenic sepsis*. Available at: https://cks.nice.org.uk/topics/neutropenic-sepsis

3. Tahir, N. and Zahra, F. (updated 2023) *Neutrophilia*. StatPearls. Available at: www.ncbi.nlm.nih.gov/books/NBK570571

4. American Cancer Society (revised 2018) *Signs and symptoms of acute myeloid leukemia (AML)*. Available at: www.cancer.org/cancer/types/acute-myeloid-leukemia/detection-diagnosis-staging/signs-symptoms.html

5. NICE (revised 2021) *Platelets – abnormal counts and cancer*. Available at: https://cks.nice.org.uk/topics/platelets-abnormal-counts-cancer

6. Bounds, E.J. and Kok, S.J. (updated 2023) *D Dimer*. StatPearls. Available at: www.ncbi.nlm.nih.gov/books/NBK431064

7. Alfonzo, A., Harrison, A., Baines, R. *et al.*, for the Renal Association (2020). *Clinical practice guidelines: treatment of acute hyperkalaemia in adults*. Available at: https://ukkidney.org/sites/renal.org/files/RENAL%20ASSOCIATION%20HYPERKALAEMIA%20GUIDELINE%20-%20JULY%202022%20V2_0.pdf

8. Castro, D. and Sharma, S. (updated 2024) *Hypokalemia*. StatPearls. Available at: www.ncbi.nlm.nih.gov/books/NBK482465

9. Liamis, G., Milionis, H.J. and Elisaf, M. (2009) A review of drug-induced hypernatraemia. *NDT Plus*, **2(5):** 339–346. Available at: www.ncbi.nlm.nih.gov/pmc/articles/PMC4421386

10. NICE (revised 2020) *Hyponatraemia*. Available at: https://cks.nice.org.uk/topics/hyponatraemia

11. NICE (revised 2024) *Chronic kidney disease*. Available at: https://cks.nice.org.uk/topics/chronic-kidney-disease

12. Hyper-/hypocalcaemia: NICE (revised 2023) *Acute kidney injury*. Available at: https://cks.nice.org.uk/topics/acute-kidney-injury

13. KDIGO (2012) *Clinical practice guideline for acute kidney injury*. Available at: https://kdigo.org/guidelines/acute-kidney-injury

14. NICE (2023) *How should I assess a person with acute kidney injury?* Available at: https://cks.nice.org.uk/topics/acute-kidney-injury/diagnosis/assessment

15. Pradhan, S., Ghimire, A., Bhattarai, B. *et al.* (2016) The role of C-reactive protein as a diagnostic predictor of sepsis in a multidisciplinary Intensive Care Unit of a tertiary care center in Nepal. *Indian J Crit Care Med*, **20(7):** 417–420. Available at: www.ncbi.nlm.nih.gov/pmc/articles/PMC4968065

27

Chapter 27: **Confirmation of life extinct**

"The greatest glory in living lies not in never falling, but in rising every time we fall."
Nelson Mandela

Who can confirm life extinct?

- In keeping with English law and contrary to popular belief, a doctor is not required to confirm death or life extinct[1].
- English law states that any competent adult can verify death; however, that person is under no obligation to do so[1].
- With regard to unexpected or sudden deaths, it is considered good practice for a doctor or a healthcare professional to attend and confirm death, thereby preventing the need for emergency services to attend.
- If death is assumed to be due to unnatural causes or has occurred in suspicious circumstances, the police should be informed immediately.
- In cases where death is expected and the patient is a resident in a residential or nursing home, verification of death can be done by a competent adult, including carers and nursing staff. The funeral directors can then be informed and the deceased can be taken away.
- If death is expected in a patient who is at home, it is good practice for a doctor to attend to confirm life extinct and provide guidance and support to the next of kin. Once life extinct has been confirmed, the funeral directors can be informed and the deceased can be taken away.
- Remote verification of death can also be undertaken, provided the doctor taking the call is confident that a competent person is present with the deceased and is capable of confirming life extinct. The competent person should be able to assess the pupils, carotid pulse and breath sounds.

Confirming life extinct

- The three findings which constitute brain death are coma (a prolonged state of unconsciousness), absence of brainstem reflexes and apnoea (the absence of spontaneous respiration)[2].
- Several conditions may mimic brain death; these include shock, hypothermia, neurogenic causes such as Guillain–Barré syndrome and myasthenia gravis, encephalitis, and overdose of neurotoxic drugs such as opiates, benzodiazepines and barbiturates[3].
- In clinical practice the absence of central pulses, heart sounds and breath sounds, along with fixed and dilated pupils, is indicative of brain death.

Issuing a medical certificate of cause of death

- Prior to the Covid-19 pandemic a medical certificate of cause of death (MCCD) could be issued by the doctor who had seen and treated the patient within the last 14 days and was able to identify a cause of death.
- In 2020 the legislation was changed to take into account the Covid-19 pandemic and as a result an MCCD could be issued by a doctor who had seen the deceased patient 28 days prior to death (including by video link) or in person, after death[4],[5].
- If these conditions are not met but the doctor is confident with regard to the cause of death, an MCCD can still be issued; however, the coroner or medical examiner should be made aware that the above conditions have not been met.
- From September 2024 NHS England introduced a new medical examiner service[6]. All deaths in any health setting that are not investigated by a coroner are reviewed by NHS medical examiners to provide independent scrutiny of deaths and to give bereaved people a voice. The MCCD can be issued by any doctor who has attended the deceased in their lifetime, in liaison with a medical examiner. The medical examiner is able to discuss the cause of death with the next of kin of the deceased, and address any concerns they have regarding care before death. It is expected that the new arrangements will provide greater safeguards, ensure referrals to the coroner are appropriate, and improve the quality of death certification and data collection.

Summary for confirmation of life extinct

- A doctor is not required to confirm death; this can be done by a competent adult.
- Remote verification can be done by a doctor, provided a competent adult can examine the deceased.
- In clinical practice the absence of central pulses, heart sounds and breath sounds, along with fixed and dilated pupils, is indicative of brain death.
- The Covid-19 pandemic in 2020 resulted in changes to legislation regarding death verification and certification.

References

1. BMA (2020) *Verification of Death (VoD), Completion of Medical Certificates of Cause of Death (MCCD) and Cremation Forms in the Community in England and Wales*. Available at: www.bma.org.uk/media/2843/bma-verification-of-death-vod-july-2020.pdf

2. Kumar, A. and Pawar, M. (2009) The diagnosis of brain death. *Indian J Crit Care Med*, **13(1):** 7–11.

3. Bhupal, H.K. (2016) *Clinical Forensic & Legal Medicine: MCQ's, answers and explanatory notes* (Death and post-mortem, pp. 49–59). CreateSpace Independent Publishing Platform.

4. RCGP & BMA Joint Guidance (2020) *Guidance for Remote Verification of Expected Death (VoED) Out of Hospital*. Available at: www.bma.org.uk/media/2323/bma-guidelines-for-remote-voed-april-2020.pdf

5. BMA (updated 2024) *COVID-19: death certification and cremation*. Available at: www.bma.org.uk/advice-and-support/covid-19/adapting-to-covid/covid-19-death-certification-and-cremation

6. NHS England (no date) *The national medical examiner system*. Available at: www.england.nhs.uk/patient-safety/medical-examiners/the-national-medical-examiner-system